PROTECTING STUDY VOLUNTEERS IN RESEARCH

A Manual for Investigative Sites

CYNTHIA MCGUIRE DUNN, M.D. & GARY CHADWICK, PHARM.D., MPH
of the University of Rochester Medical Center

CenterWatch, Inc.
22 Thomson Place, 12F3 • Boston, MA 02210-1212
(617) 856-5900 (Phone) • (617) 856-5901 (Fax)
www.centerwatch.com
A Medical Economics Company

To purchase additional copies of this manual, please call (800) 765-9647

CenterWatch Book Editor: Whitney Allen
CenterWatch Publisher: Ken Getz
Design and Production: Innovative Printing Group

FOREWORD

As demand for new technology and knowledge increases, research has become more complex. The science, design and conduct of research have all changed dramatically since the human subject protection regulations were consolidated in 1981. Studies are exploring areas only vaguely conceptualized two decades ago. The number and diversity of human subjects involved in studies are increasing.

Consequently, the ethical considerations associated with research have become more complex. To keep the public's trust, the research community must effectively protect human subjects while allowing appropriate access. All members of the research community have a responsibility to ensure that research is conducted ethically. Rigorous compliance with ethical standards and practices will also promote scientific discovery.

Violations in research ethics are generally caused by lack of awareness rather than malice. Although common sense is valuable, research does present unique circumstances and special considerations. The importance of training for researchers cannot be over-stressed. If all researchers were well-versed in ethics and complied with regulations, institutional review boards and other oversight mechanisms would not be as necessary. Researchers do not need to be regulatory experts, but they do need a certain level of knowledge about these issues. They need to know and understand a few basic requirements and the underlying ethical principles.

The intent of this manual is to aid researchers in understanding the regulatory requirements and ethical principles upon which they are based. The manual will also identify issues that require sensitivity when designing or conducting human research studies. Ultimately the safety and welfare of human subjects rests in the hands of the investigators. We hope this manual will aid all members of the research community in promoting ethical scientific discovery.

– CMD

– GLC

ACKNOWLEDGEMENTS

Manual Development Coordination:

Judith R. Farrar, Ph.D.
Director
Academic Services Consortium

Jeanine Smith, M.S., CCRA
Associate Director
Academic Services Consortium

Additional Authors (University of Rochester):

Christine Burke, J.D.
Deputy Counsel
University of Rochester Medical Center

Joanne C. Larson, Ph.D.
Assistant Professor
Warner Graduate School of
Education and Development

Timothy Hackett
Manager of Quality Assurance
Clinical Research Institute

Rebecca Thom, Ph.D.
Director, Industry Affairs
Research Subjects Review Board

William Kelvie, CCRC
Director, Clinical Research Practices
Clinical Research Institute

Gunta Liders
Associate Director
Research and Project Administration

Advisory Review Committee:

Peggy Cunningham, B.S.N., M.S.
Roche Labs, Inc.

Dale W. McAdam, Ph.D.
University of Rochester

David Forster, J.D., M.A.
Western Institutional Review Board

Harold Vanderpool, Ph.D., Th.M.
University of Texas Medical Branch

Jeanne Grace, R.N.C., Ph.D.
University of Rochester

Karen Woodin, Ph.D.
ClinTrials Research, Inc.

Robert Levine, M.D.
Yale University School of Medicine

Gary Yingling, J.D.
McKenna & Cuneo

Louis Lasagna, M.D.
Tufts University

TABLE OF CONTENTS

Instructions For Obtaining Continuing Education Credit i

Chapter One: Historical Perspectives on Human Subject Research 1
Introduction 1
The Nuremberg Doctors Trial of 1946 2
The 'Milgram Study' 5
Thalidomide Tragedy. 7
The Study of Untreated Syphilis In The Negro Male 8
Human Radiation Experiments. 11
Conclusion. 13

Chapter Two: Ethics and Federal Regulations. 15
Introduction 15
Belmont Report. 16
Basic Principles of Belmont Report. 16
Federal Regulations 24

Chapter Three: The Roles and Responsibilities of Institutions in Human Subject Research. . . 33
Introduction 33
Research Institution 33
Federal Agencies. 37
Good Clinical Practice (GCP). 38

Chapter Four: The Roles and Responsibilities of the Investigator and The Study Process . . . 41
Introduction 41
Investigator's Role and Responsibilities. 42
Research Team Roles and Responsibilities. 45
Study Process. 46

Chapter Five: FDA-Regulated Research Issues 57
Introduction 57
Drugs and Biologics/INDs 58
Medical Devices/IDEs 59
Sponsor Responsibilities in FDA-Regulated Research. 60
The Study Process for Industry-Sponsored Studies. 62
Sponsor-Investigator-Institution Interaction Issues. 67
Responsibilities of The Investigator-Sponsor 67

Chapter Six: Behavioral Research Issues 73
Introduction 73
Federal Regulations 73
Psychological/Social Risks 74

TABLE OF CONTENTS (continued)

Deception 75
Vulnerable Subjects 76
Privacy and Confidentiality 76
Study Methods.. 77
Quality of Life Issues... 77
Points to Consider 78

Chapter Seven: Publication of Study Results **79**
Introduction 79
Withholding Data 85
Lessons to be Learned From These Cases 86
The Data.. 87
Summary.. 88

APPENDIX

Appendix A: References, Resources and Suggested Readings................... **91**

Appendix B: The Belmont Report **95**

Appendix C: Code of Federal Regulations................................ **109**

Appendix D: Glossary.. **215**

Appendix E: Abbreviations... **221**

Index.. **223**

Examination Questions **225**

INSTRUCTIONS FOR OBTAINING CONTINUING EDUCATION CREDIT

How to use the Manual:

In an effort to make this manual as relevant to your work as possible, we have focused on topics, regulations and guidelines that are most pertinent to academic research. This manual does not include specific code references to the regulations, nor does it provide sample documents. While some of the regulations are included in the appendix, both the regulation codes and documents are subject to change. Specific resources that can provide additional information are provided in the References, Resources, and Suggested Reading section of the appendix. Also, remember to contact your institutional review board (IRB) with any questions and for regular updates on relevant regulations and documents.

Certification

For Physicians:

The University of Rochester School of Medicine and Dentistry adheres to the Accreditation Council for Continuing Medical Education (ACCME) standards regarding industry support of continuing medical education.

This continuing education activity was planned and produced in accordance with the Essentials and Standards of ACCME.

The University of Rochester School of Medicine and Dentistry is accredited by ACCME to sponsor continuing medical education for physicians. The University of Rochester School of Medicine and Dentistry takes responsibility for the content, quality and scientific integrity of this CME activity.

The University of Rochester School of Medicine and Dentistry designates this educational activity for up to 4.0 hours in Category 1 credit toward the AMA Physician's Recognition Award. Each physician should claim only those hours of credit that he/she actually spent in the educational activity.

Category 1 credit valid through June 30, 2002.

For Nurses:

This activity has also been approved by the New York State Nurses Association's Council on Continuing Education, which is accredited by the American Nurses Credentialing Center's Commission on Accreditation, and is assigned approval code UNIVROCH1-5282-99. This has been assigned 4.8 contact hours.

Nursing contact hours valid through April 22, 2001.

To obtain credit:

1. Read the manual.

2. Answer the exam questions on the answer sheet provided. Questions and answers are based on information in the manual. Participants who answer 85% of the questions correctly will receive up to 4.0 hours of continuing medical education credit or 4.8 nursing contact hours.

3. Complete the evaluation questions on the <u>Protecting Study Volunteers in Research</u> evaluation form. **Note! Credit can not be issued if the evaluation form is not received with the answer sheet.**

4. Complete the mailing information portion of the answer sheet.

5. Detach and mail the answer sheet and evaluation form by June 30, 2002 for CME credits, and by April 22, 2001 for nursing contact hours.

University of Rochester School of Medicine and Dentistry
Office of Continuing Professional Education
601 Elmwood Avenue, Box 677
Rochester, NY 14642-8677

6. You will receive a certificate in the mail within two to four weeks.

7. Call (716) 275-4392 with questions or for further information.

Please take the time to carefully read this Manual. We hope that you will regularly refer to it as a guide for your studies involving human research subjects.

1

HISTORICAL PERSPECTIVES ON HUMAN SUBJECT RESEARCH

Objectives

At the conclusion of this chapter, readers will be able to:

- Describe three events that had significant impact on the federal regulations for the protection of the human research subjects.

- Have a better understanding of why we need compliance regulations and how compliance helps protect the rights and welfare of human research subjects.

Introduction

History is not static. Yesterday's actions are today's history. The public's perception of research, its benefits and its risks are shaped by the way research is conducted. Recent events have renewed concerns about research ethics. Included are issues regarding informed consent with incapacitated subjects (TD v. New York State) and responsibilities of researchers for subject welfare (after the death of a student volunteer in a research study at Rochester and the suicide of a schizophrenic subject during a study 'washout period' at UCLA). In the United States, concerns such as these often result in government action affecting the conduct and monitoring of research.*

---

*Recent examples are the congressional General Accounting Office (GAO) Report on Human Subject Research (1994); The Department of Health and Human Services (DHHS) Report on Institutional Review Boards (1998); Research Involving Subjects with Disorders that may Affect Decision-making Capacity: a draft report of the President's National Bioethics Advisory Commission (NBAC); Third Report of the [Maryland] Attorney General's Research Working Group; and the 1998 New York State Department of Health (NYS-DH) report on human subjects in research.

> The public's perception of research, its benefits and its risks is shaped by the way research is conducted.

Historically, there are three events that have had significant impact on federal regulations for the protection of human research subjects. In chronological order, these are the 1946 Nuremberg Doctors Trial, the 1960s Thalidomide Tragedy and the 1972 Tuskegee Syphilis Study Exposé. While other events such as the Willowbrook Studies, the Wichita Jury Study, the Jewish Chronic Disease Hospital Study and the San Antonio Contraceptive Study also played a role, the cases discussed below had the most direct impact on shaping federal regulations. One additional case, the Milgram Study, will be reviewed. While it did not have the same scope or impact on federal regulations, this study is included because it is often cited in ethics literature as illustrative of potential problems in behavioral research. Also presented is the 1995 report on Human Radiation Experiments that measured how well the regulations are working.

The Nuremberg Doctors Trial of 1946

Background

At the beginning of World War II, Germany was the most scientifically and technologically advanced country in the world and even had a proposed code of research ethics. In the field of medicine, the Nazi government supported midwifery, homeopathy and nutrition programs as well as research into ecology, public health, human genetics, cancer, radiation and asbestos. They were the first to ban smoking in public buildings. Women were denied tobacco ration coupons because of concern about the effect of nicotine on the fetus. German physicians stressed the importance of preventive medicine rather than curative medicine. The Nazis, however, exploited people's trust in physicians to disguise discrimination and murder as public health.

Medical Experiments

A legitimate concern of the German Air Force was the survival of pilots at extremely high altitudes and determining the maximum safe altitude for bailing out of damaged aircraft. In one series of experiments, researchers placed victims in vacuum chambers that could duplicate the low air pressure and lack of oxygen at altitudes as high as 65,000 feet (about two to three times the maximum altitude that aircraft were flying). Approximately 200 internees at Dachau were used in these experiments, and about 40% died as a result. Some deaths were caused by extended anoxia; others were attributable to lungs rupturing from the low pressures in the chamber.

Another concern was survival time after parachuting into the cold water of the North Atlantic. Some victims of this research were immersed for hours in tubs of ice water; others were fed nothing but salt water for days. Still others were penned outside, unclothed and unsheltered in sub-freezing temperatures for 12 to 14 hours. Some of these "freezing victims" were sprayed with cold water. No attempts were made to relieve the tremendous pain and suffering caused by these experiments. Three hundred Dachau prisoner-subjects suffered a mortality rate of about 30%.

Experiments involving battlefield medicine included treatment of gunshot wounds, burns, traumatic amputations and chemical and biological agent exposures. In these experiments, the wound was first inflicted upon the victim (by gunshot, stabbing, amputation or other traumatic method) and then treated using various techniques. For example, in a study of sulfanilamide at the Ravensbrueck camp, Polish women were shot and slashed on the legs. The resulting wounds were stuffed with glass, dirt and various bacteria cultures, and sewn shut. The infected wounds were then treated with experimental anti-infective agents. In another experiment, a mixture of phosphorus and rubber was applied to the skin of victims and ignited. After burning for up to two minutes, the fire was extinguished and the resultant burn treated with various chemicals and ointments. Another series of experiments involved amputation of upper and lower limbs, and attempted treatment with transplanted bones, muscle and nerves. Neither the victim nor the tissue 'donor' did well in these studies: about half of the amputation victims died, the rest were maimed for life.

Experiments on treating exposure to chemical-warfare agents were ongoing throughout the war years. Prisoners were forced to drink poisoned water and breathe noxious gases. Some were shot with cyanide-tipped bullets or given cyanide capsules. A mortality rate of 25% was typical.

The Nuremberg Trial

On August 8, 1945, representatives of the British, French, Soviet and United States governments established the International Military Tribunal in Nuremberg, Germany. After the initial Nuremberg Trial of the Nazi leadership, a series of supplemental trials was held. The trial, officially known as United States v. Karl Brandt et al., and popularly referred to as "The Nazi Doctors Trial," was held from December 9, 1946 to August 20, 1947. As the title indicates, for this trial, the judges and prosecutors were all from the United States. The 23 defendants (including 20 physicians) were charged with murder, torture and other atrocities committed in the name of medical science.

When the Nazi Doctors Trial was completed on August 20, 1947, 15 of the 23 defendants were found guilty. Seven were sentenced to death. Although the trial was called "The Trial of the Century," it would probably have been forgotten except for the fact that the judgment included a set of standards known as the Nuremberg Code. The Code, was the 'ethical yardstick' by which the defendants had been measured and guilt determined. The 'Modern' era of human subject protection is routinely dated from the promulgation of the Nuremberg Code.

The Code stated, that:

- Informed consent of volunteers must be obtained without coercion in any form.

- Human experiments should be based upon prior animal experimentation.

- Anticipated scientific results should justify the experiment.

- Only qualified scientists should conduct medical research.

- Physical and mental suffering and injury should be avoided.

- There should be no expectation of death or disabling injury from the experiment.

> The 'Modern' era of human subject protection is routinely dated from the promulgation of the Nuremberg Code in 1947.

Post-war Years

In 1953, the World Medical Association began drafting a document that became known as the Declaration of Helsinki. This statement of ethical principles, first issued in 1964, defined rules for 'therapeutic' and 'non-therapeutic' research. It repeated the Nuremberg Code requirement for consent for non-therapeutic research, but it did allow for enrolling certain patients in therapeutic research without consent. The Declaration of Helsinki also allowed legal guardians to grant permission to enroll subjects in research, both therapeutic and non-therapeutic. Several revisions have been made to the Declaration of Helsinki to keep it aligned with modern ethical theory and current clinical and research practices.

In 1966, following the publication of the Declaration of Helsinki, Dr. Henry K. Beecher reported in the *New England Journal of Medicine*

(NEJM) on 22 studies that had serious ethical problems. Beecher cited various problems related to study design and to informed consent. Probably even more than the Nuremberg Trial/Code, this article (and his other earlier publications) helped to spur the debate on research ethics in this country.

In 1982, The Council for the International Organization of Medical Sciences (CIOMS) published the International Ethics Guidelines for Biomedical Research Involving Human Subjects (CIOMS Guidelines). These were designed to guide researchers from the more technologically advanced countries when conducting research in developing countries. The guideline sought to correct perceived omissions in the Nuremburg Code and Declaration of Helsinki, especially as applied to cross-cultural research. The CIOMS Guidelines allow for cultural differences in ethical standards.

The 'Milgram Study'

Background

Stanley Milgram was a researcher in social psychology who, after reading accounts of the Nazi Holocaust, became interested in obedience and humans' response to authority. The German citizenry's seeming acceptance of and complacency in regard to the atrocities presented an interesting question. In 1963, he published the results of a study on obedience that raised a firestorm of criticism with implications even today.

The Experiment

Adult subjects were recruited by means of a newspaper advertisement asking for volunteers for a study of 'memory and learning.' Participants were paid a modest amount for the one hour experiment. Study participants were part of a triad that consisted of themselves, the investigator and a third person. The investigator explained that the experiment was to study learning and memory, specifically what role punishment played. The subject was to play the role of 'teacher' while the third person was to be the 'learner.' The investigator would monitor the process and record the data.

The learner was placed in what appeared to be an electric chair, that is, wire leads ran from a control panel to the chair and were attached to the learner's wrists. The control panel had switches labeled from 15 volts to 450 volts.

For the experiment, the subject-teacher asked the learner a question (word-pair matching) and when the wrong answer was given, the investigator would instruct the subject to administer 'punishment' to the learner in the form of electric shocks in an escalating amount. The learner would display evidence of receiving pain from the shocks. After one-third of the shock levels had been given, the learner demanded to stop. At this point, the subject-teacher would usually ask the investigator to stop, but the investigator insisted that the procedure continue. After two thirds of the shocks had been administered, the learner fell silent and non-responsive (a non-response was treated as a wrong answer and punished). When they continued to seek permission to stop, the highly conflicted subject-teachers were told that the experiment was important to complete for the advancement of science. Fully 60% of subject-teachers were persuaded into administering shocks up to and including the highest level.

What the subjects did not know was that the third person who played the role of learner was in fact a confederate of the investigator. No shocks were administered. The learner (who deliberately gave wrong answers) only pretended to be hurt. The real intent of the experiment was to see how far the subject could be pushed under the guise of complying with authority. At the completion of the experiment (either after the maximum shock was ostensibly given or upon firm refusal by the subject to continue), the confederate came out of his room and demonstrated to the subject that he was uninjured. A debriefing with the subject was held that explained the deception and the real purpose of the study. During the debriefing interviews, subjects often justified their actions by saying that they were only following instructions. (A similar line was taken by the Nazi defendants.)

> *"I observed a mature and initially poised businessman enter the laboratory smiling and confident. Within twenty minutes he was reduced to a twitching, stuttering wreck, who was rapidly approaching a point of nervous collapse."*
>
> Stanley Milgram in *Obedience to Authority*

Impact

Criticism of the study centered upon the extreme psychological stress experienced by some subjects and on the fact that due to the deception involved, informed consent had not been obtained. The role of deception in human subject research continues to be debated even today. Ethical codes such as the Nuremberg Code and the Declaration of Helsinki point to the importance of obtaining consent that is informed, understood and voluntary. Common sense and experience tell us that people act differently when they know they are being studied. The federal regulations specifically allow for deception in research, but only in limited conditions and only with IRB approval.

> When deception is involved, true informed consent cannot be obtained.

As a result of this and other behavioral studies, the federal guidelines specifically instruct investigators and IRBs to consider not just physical harms that may be attached to research, but also other harms including psychological, social, legal and economic.

Thalidomide Tragedy

Background

Thalidomide was approved as a sedative in Europe in the late 1950s. Although the U.S. Food and Drug Administration (FDA) had not approved the drug, the manufacturer supplied 'samples' to U. S. physicians who were paid to study its safety and efficacy in what was loosely termed "research" by giving the experimental drug to patients. This was a common practice of pharmaceutical companies at that time. By 1961, experience in Europe, Canada and, to a lesser extent, in this country, showed that while thalidomide was not harmful to the mother, it was extremely damaging to the fetus if taken in the first trimester of pregnancy. It interfered with the normal development of arms and legs. Based upon its teratogenicity, use of the drug as a sedative was banned world-wide.

Thalidomide Hearings and their Impact

A U.S. Senate subcommittee, chaired by Senator Hubert Humphrey, heard testimony about the thalidomide disaster, which was receiving extensive coverage in the news media. The pictures of deformed and limbless babies raised questions about the procedures used to test experimental drugs. It was learned that many people who were taking the drug were neither informed that they were being given an experimental substance, nor had they been asked to give their consent. Another subcommittee chaired by Senator Estes Kefauver had been holding hearings (1959 - 1962) into the business practices of pharmaceutical companies. The public concern over research practices addressed in these two committees lead to the passage of the Drug Amendments of 1962 to the Food, Drug and Cosmetic Act (sometimes referred to as the Kefauver-Harris Amendments, as the bill was drafted by their Antitrust and Monopoly subcommittee). New York Senator Jacob Javits added language to the bill that required informed consent of subjects receiving experimental drugs. This was the first U.S. statute that required researchers to inform subjects of a drug's experimental nature and to receive their consent before starting the research.

In February 1963, the FDA issued regulations with a consent requirement but they allowed widespread exemption. Responding to concerns that consent was still not being appropriately obtained, in 1966, the regulations were rewritten to clarify that consent was required except in cases of emergency or experimental therapeutic treatments with children and similar situations. The 1966 rewrite also contained the requirement for documenting consent in writing and informing subjects that they might receive a placebo.

The Study of Untreated Syphilis in the Negro Male

Background

The treatment for syphilis at the turn of the twentieth century was, at best, crude and involved the use of 'heavy metal' (mercury and arsenic) compounds. These were poisons, highly toxic to humans, and had to be administered for a year or more. Severe reactions, even death, were not uncommon from the treatment and some evidence suggested that treated patients lived shorter lives than the untreated.

An agency of the U.S. Public Health Service (PHS), which was to become the Centers for Disease Control and Prevention (CDC), designed a study to demonstrate the need for establishing syphilis treatment programs by investigating the effects of untreated disease. This evolved from a genuine concern about minority health problems. The PHS was a key force in promoting rural medical care. Macon County, Alabama, was selected as the site for the project because previous epidemiological studies had shown an extremely high rate of disease. Thus began the Tuskegee Study of Untreated Syphilis in the Negro Male.* To secure the cooperation of the black subjects, the participation of black physicians was seen as essential. The Tuskegee Institute and its John A. Andrew Hospital were used because of their position of trust in the local community. A local nurse who had trained at the Tuskegee Institute was hired to be the on-site representative. The project was scheduled to end after assessing what health effects had occurred.

---

* The Tuskegee Study of Untreated Syphilis in the Negro Male has been most commonly called the Tuskegee Study. Due to concern for the negative connotations for the Tuskegee Institute, some are calling for a change in the shorthand name. Therefore, this manual will use the term "The Syphilis Study."

In the beginning, there was no intent to deny anyone treatment on a long-term basis. The study called for 200 to 300 syphilitic black males, aged 25 and older, to be enrolled. They were to be given complete physical examinations, a thorough medical history and then followed for six to eight months. During that time, they would not be treated. This study demonstrates that competent and well-intentioned researchers may run into problems unless regular re-examination and consideration of ethical concerns occurs.

The Experiment

In October 1932, subjects were sought and encouraged to participate in the study with offers of free examinations and medical care. The men were not informed about their disease or the fact that the research would not benefit them. Non-therapeutic spinal taps, which were conducted in May 1933, were supposed to end the experiment; but a second phase of study started in late 1933. This phase introduced new procedures to strengthen scientific validity and to gain more information. A control group of 200 black men and autopsies of deceased subjects were added to the study. Like the original subjects, the members of the control group were not informed about the purpose of the study, but were told that 'government doctors' were examining people for 'bad blood.'

Each year, new physicians were sent on special assignment to Alabama to conduct the 'roundups' and medical examinations. The study procedures became so routine that the study continued without any exploration or understanding of the potential ramifications of the project. Many of the itinerant physicians later filled positions of authority in the PHS and/or CDC.

In 1943, penicillin was accepted as the treatment for syphilis. However, during World War II, to keep the syphilis subjects from receiving treatment, it was arranged with the local draft board to exempt them from the military. By 1951, penicillin was widely available as the treatment for syphilis, but it continued to be withheld from the study subjects.

Actually, the availability of penicillin was used by the study investigators as justification for continuing the study because it made the protocol a 'never-again' scientific opportunity. Neither the ethical issues nor the fact that the supposedly untreated subjects had received some minimal treatment were addressed. No connection was made between the Syphilis Study and the Nazi experiments. Announcement of the

Nuremberg Code had no impact on the study.

Exposé

After obtaining copies of letters and other study-related documents in 1972, the Associated Press assigned an investigative reporter, Jean Heller to uncover the story. Her best source of information was the CDC itself. The study had never been hidden, several articles had been published and CDC officials discussed it candidly. Her story was published in the *New York Times* and the *Washington Star* on July 25, 1972.

The public reaction to the Syphilis Study was strong. James B. Allen, a U.S. Senator from Alabama, denounced the study as appalling, "a disgrace to the American concept of justice and humanity." The fact that the PHS had conducted the study was particularly distressing because instead of protecting citizens, it had used them for research. Some people thought that the study was racist. Others believed that social class was the critical issue, i.e., that poor people, regardless of race were the ones at risk because they made up a disproportionate share of subjects in most medical experiments.

An article that appeared in the *Atlanta Constitution* on July 27, 1972, stated, "Sometimes, with the best of intentions, scientists and public officials and others involved in working for the benefit of us all, forget that people are people. They concentrate so totally on plans and programs, experiments, statistics - on abstractions - that people become objects, symbols on paper, figures in a mathematical formula or impersonal 'subjects' in a scientific study." Many saw a need to protect people from experiments and scientists who ignored human values.

In reaction to the revelations about the Syphilis Study and other research 'scandals', several bills to regulate research were introduced in Congress. During February and March 1973, Senator Edward Kennedy held hearings on experimentation with human subjects. In March 1973, the Syphilis Study was stopped, and treatment was given as needed. In April 1973, the CDC informed the survivors that the government would pay all of their medical expenses for the rest of their lives. In 1975, the government extended treatment to the wives who had contracted syphilis and to their children who had been born with congenital syphilis. This money continues to be paid today. In a formal White House ceremony in 1997, President Clinton apologized to study subjects and their families and called for renewed emphasis on research ethics.

In 1974, Congress passed the National Research Act. The Act required regulations for the protection of human subjects that included requirements for informed consent and review of research by institutional review boards (IRBs). This Act also created the National Commission for the Protection of Human Subjects of Biomedical and Behavioral Research. In 1979, the National Commission wrote the "Belmont Report," which is the cornerstone statement of ethical principles upon which the federal regulations for the protection of subjects are based.

In 1981, the DHHS and the FDA published convergent regulations that were based on the Belmont Principles. These mandated a role on the IRB for persons with broad backgrounds and members who could represent community attitudes. Informed consent was required for participants and specific elements of information were listed. After 10 years of negotiation and coordination, 17 federal departments and agencies agreed to adopt the basic human subject protections. These were published in 1991 and are referred to as the 'Common Rule.' Thus, essentially all federally sponsored research is now covered by a common set of regulations that has its origins in the National Research Act and the Syphilis Study.

Human Radiation Experiments

Background

In November 1993, the Albuquerque Tribune published a series of articles by Eileen Welsome that revealed that, under government sponsorship, researchers at several major universities had injected plutonium into unknowing subjects to study the effects of the atomic bomb. That same month, a congressional report described 13 cases in which nuclear facilities had intentionally released radiation into the environment for government experiments.

These revelations raised concern about the adequacy of protection provided by federal laws and regulations. In January 1994, President Clinton created the Advisory Committee on Human Radiation Experiments (ACHRE) to explore human radiation experiments and to determine what the ethical and scientific standards were for evaluating these events. When he accepted the Committee's Final Report in 1995, President Clinton ordered the creation of the National Bioethics Advisory Commission (NBAC), which continues to refine thinking on human experimentation and to make recommendations on the regulation of research.

Experiments

The ACHRE discovered that several thousand government-sponsored human radiation experiments and hundreds of intentional releases of radiation from nuclear facilities were conducted from 1944 to 1974. Most of the radiation experiments involved low risk uses of radioisotopes in legitimate biomedical research. However, other experiments were not so benign.

The 'Manhattan Project' plutonium injection experiments were conducted for national security and to gather safety data to protect the health and safety of nuclear weapons workers. The results are still used in the nuclear industry today. In one series of experiments, over one 100 prisoners submitted to non-therapeutic testicular irradiation. Up to 3,000 military personnel served as subjects of research in connection with atomic bomb tests, sometimes unknowingly. About 2,000 cancer patients were subjected to total body irradiation strictly to find answers to problems in the development and use of atomic weapons. A review conducted by the Atomic Energy Commission (AEC) in 1974 found that while 18 subjects were given plutonium injections between the years 1945 and 1947, the records documented only one subject's consent.

Eighty-one examples of pediatric radiation research projects were identified by the ACHRE. Fortunately, although children are more susceptible than adults to harm from low levels of radiation, the exposures to radiation were very low and probably did not pose a risk of physical harm.

Response

In addition to exploring the case studies summarized above, the ACHRE Report discussed the historical development of research ethics and examined issues related to implementing and interpreting current federal regulations. The ACHRE's most serious concerns about current practices focused on informed consent. Some contemporary consent documents were found to be difficult to read, uninformative, and even misleading. Informed consent was particularly troubling in research involving patient-subjects with poor prognoses because these patients are so vulnerable, and are often confused about the relationship of research to treatment. There also was concern about the inappropriate use of the word 'treatment' in consent forms, especially in phase 1 trials of new drugs.

The ACHRE found that, when compared to the information in the grant proposal and/or protocol, consent forms often overstated the benefits and therapeutic potential of the research. Such overstatements may inappropriately induce enrollment by playing on the hopes of patients or on the philanthropy of volunteers. The review also showed that consent forms did not always discuss the risks that subjects faced when removed from standard treatment in order to be placed on experimental interventions. There often was little mention of how participation would affect the subject's daily life or the quality of life. Psycho-social risks were often inadequately addressed in proposal documents, as were potential financial costs that could be incurred.

The final portion of the report included recommendations to better ensure that those who conduct research involving human subjects act in a manner consistent with the interests and rights of subjects, and consistent with the highest standards of medical and scientific ethics. The recommendations stated that it is essential that the research community come to value the ethics of research as central to the scientific process. Because the future of science depends to a great extent upon public support and public trust, scientists must have a clear understanding of their duties to human subjects and scientific leaders must value good ethics as much as they do good science. The ACHRE's call for making ethics the center piece of the research enterprise and recommending increased training in research ethics may be the most important step in the continuing evolution of human subject protections.

> *"It is essential that the research community come to value the ethics of research as central to the scientific process."*
>
> National Bioethics Advisory Commission

Conclusion

Investigators bear the ultimate ethical responsibility for their work with human subjects. Society entrusts them with the privilege of using other humans to advance scientific knowledge. In return, society expects that investigators will show respect for research subjects. Unfortunately, as events have shown, some scientists still continue to value the quest for knowledge more highly than respect for basic human rights. The research community as a whole suffers when even a few investigators ignore basic principles of ethics. Compliance with human subject protection regulations should not be seen as something that must be done just because it is required by the regulations. Compliance should be seen as the 'right thing to do' because it helps protect the rights and welfare of the subjects of human research.

Research Ethics Milestones

National Bioethics Advisory Commission __1995__

Common Rule __1991__

CIOMS Guidelines __1982__

Consolidated HHS/FDA Regulations __1981__

Belmont Report __1979__

_ _ . _ . _The Syphilis Study (Exposé)

Declaration of Helsinki 1964

_ 1966 _The Beecher Article (NEJM)

Kefauver-Harris Amendments to the __1962__ Food, Drug and Cosmetic Act

_ . _ . _ . _ . _ . _Milgram Study

Trigger Events

_ . _ . _ . _ . _ . _The Thalidomide Tragedy

Nuremberg __1947__ Code

_ . _ . _ . _ . _ . _Human Radiation Experiments

_ . _ . _ . _ . _ . _The Nazi Experiments

_ . _ . _ _The Syphilis Study (Begins)

CHAPTER 2

ETHICS AND FEDERAL REGULATIONS

Objectives

At the conclusion of this chapter, readers will be able to:

- Describe the relevance of the Belmont Report on federal regulations protecting human subjects in research.

- Identify what populations are considered vulnerable, and develop an awareness of circumstances requiring sensitivity.

- Define informed consent and describe the three components of valid informed consent.

- Describe the requirements for an Institutional Assurance of Compliance.

- Describe the purpose and function of the Institutional Review Board (IRB).

- Define scientific misconduct and describe how it is reported.

Introduction

The ethics of human subject research and the federal regulations have evolved over the past 40 years. Professional associations and international organizations have also developed codes of ethics that cover research with human subjects. This chapter (and in fact, the whole manual) emphasizes the federal regulations because they are seen as a standard for the conduct of research. Compliance with the requirements of the federal regulations, even for non-federally sponsored/regulated research, protects the rights and welfare of subjects. Most institutions with Multiple Project Assurances require compliance with federal regulations for all studies regardless of source of support.

Belmont Report

In 1974, Congress passed the National Research Act. The Act created the National Commission for the Protection of Human Subjects of Biomedical and Behavioral Research. The National Commission wrote the Ethical Principles and Guidelines for the Protection of Human Subjects of Research (commonly called the Belmont Report), which was published in the Federal Register in 1979. This document is the cornerstone statement of ethical principles upon which the federal regulations for the protection of subjects are based. A copy of the Belmont Report is included in the appendix.

> The Belmont Report contains the ethical principles upon which the federal regulations for protection of human subjects are based.

Scientific research has produced substantial societal benefits. It has also posed some troubling ethical questions. Public attention was drawn to these questions by reported abuses of human subjects in scientific experiments. As a result, national and state laws and regulations, as well as international and professional codes, have been developed to guide investigators. Such rules are based upon broader ethical principles that provide an analytical framework to evaluate human actions. The Belmont Report described three basic principles relevant to the ethics of human subject research: respect for persons, beneficence and justice.

**Basic Principles of
The Belmont Report**

1. Respect for Persons

2. Beneficence

3. Justice

16

1. Respect for Persons

Respect for persons incorporates two ethical convictions: first, that individuals should be treated as autonomous agents; and second, that persons with diminished autonomy are entitled to increased protection. The principle of respect for persons thus includes two separate moral requirements: the requirement to acknowledge autonomy and the requirement to protect those with diminished autonomy.

> The principle of respect for persons is captured in the consent process.

Vulnerable Subjects

By definition, 'vulnerable populations' are those groups that may contain some individuals who have limited autonomy (i.e., they cannot fully participate in the consent process). Such groups include children, some mentally disabled, individuals with dementia and other cognitive disorders and prisoners. Special considerations apply when conducting research with these populations. Pregnant women are also recognized by the regulations as a vulnerable population because of the additional health concerns during pregnancy and because of the need to avoid unnecessary risk to the fetus.

> Vulnerable populations include some individuals who have limited autonomy such that they cannot fully participate in the consent process.

Prisoners

The regulations for human subject protection make special provisions pertaining to research with prison populations. The incarcerated may be at greater risk for coercion. Special considerations for prison studies include ensuring that:

- Any potential advantages to the prisoner for participating do not interfere with the ability to make a voluntary choice by outweighing the risks (e.g., parole decisions will not be affected by study participation).

- The risks of participating would be acceptable to non-prisoner volunteers.

- Selection of subjects within the prison system is fair.

- Adequate follow-up care is provided, if necessary.

Children

Legally, children have not attained the age where they can grant consent for research or treatment. Additional regulatory protections are established for research with children. Under these regulations, some of the exempt categories are deemed to be not applicable to research with children. Research that would be exempt for adults but not for children includes the use of survey, questionnaire or interview procedures and participatory observation. This is because a child's responses are less guarded than an adult's, and information may be divulged inappropriately.

Consent cannot be given by another person. Only an individual can provide consent for oneself. Parents or guardians, however, may provide "permission" for their child to participate in a research study. Children should be asked about their willingness or "assent" to participate. Information about the research study must be presented to children on their level, so they can understand what is requested of them. The combination of "assent" (agreement) of the minor subject and "permission" of the parent or legal guardian is generally deemed an adequate substitute for consent.

Adequate provision must be made for soliciting the assent of those children capable of providing a meaningful agreement. The process must be appropriate to the study as well as to the age, maturity and psychological state of the child. An exception to the assent requirement is made for children with life-threatening illnesses who are entered into "open-label treatment protocols" with the expectation of direct benefit. In these cases, the permission of the parent is sufficient, but the understanding of the minor subject is still desirable.

Documentation of the minor-subject's assent and the parents' permission also depends upon the nature of the research and the maturity of the child. For research with very young children (pre-school and under), only the parent's permission form is typically needed. For older adolescents, a single form that both the minor and the parent(s) sign may be adequate. For children in between (e.g., ages seven to 14), two forms are generally advisable: one written at a basic level for the child (as a "script" for oral presentation or for reading), and a more detailed form for the parent's understanding and signature.

Research in schools: In addition to the federal children's regulations, investigators who do research in schools should be aware of laws governing the conduct of these studies and disclosure of information. Two laws, FERPA (Family Educational Rights and Privacy Act) and PPRA

(Protection of Pupil Rights Amendment) apply to research in schools.

FERPA defines the rights of students and parents concerning reviewing, amending and disclosing education records. Except under certain circumstances involving treatment, order of subpoena educational or financial aid, FERPA requires that written permission must be obtained to disclose personally identifiable information from a student's educational records. Researchers who wish to inspect student records must obtain parental permission if identifiers are linked to the data.

Survey research in schools is regulated under PPRA. This law states that surveys, questionnaires and instructional materials can be inspected by parents or guardians; and parental permission must be obtained to allow minors to participate in a survey revealing information concerning the following:

- Political affiliations.

- Mental and psychological problems.

- Income.

- Sex behavior and attitudes.

- Illegal, anti-social, self-incriminating and demeaning behavior.

- Critical appraisals of other individuals with close family relationships.

- Legally recognized, privileged relationships (e.g., lawyers, physicians, ministers).

Subordinate Individuals

College students, employees and other persons in subordinate positions or positions of lesser power/status provide an easily accessible group with the potential for undue influence to impede free choice in the consent process. Employees must not be pressured to participate in research due to fear of job loss, delayed promotion or other influence of a superior. For student subjects, investigators need to consider the following:

- If course credit is given for participation, alternatives for receiving equal credit that are no more burdensome than the participation in research.

- Policies regarding course-related research participation must be clearly understood.

- Incentives for participation may not be unduly influencing.

- Student subjects must have the ability to decline participation.

- Confidentiality must be maintained for self-disclosures of a personal nature.

Decisionally Impaired

The regulations for human subjects protection do not yet make special provisions for persons whose mental status is impaired. This vulnerable population may include persons with psychiatric illness, neurologic conditions, substance use and various metabolic disorders. The level of impairment may range from poor judgment to frank coma. The National Bioethics Advisory Commission (NBAC) and several states are examining the issue and have published recommendations and suggested rules.

Until federal regulations are adopted, most investigators and IRBs use a combination of special protections gathered from the DHHS regulations for children and prisoners. As with children, some individuals in this group may not be able to give informed consent. A combination of "permission" from legally authorized representatives and the "assent" of subjects to participate are substituted for consent. Witnesses, periodic re-consent and formal checks of comprehension may be included as additional protections. Special considerations for studies in this population include ensuring that:

- The risks of participating would be acceptable to volunteers in the general public.

- Selection of subjects is fair.

- The consent information is understandable given the expected level of function.

- Adequate follow-up is provided.

Informed Consent

The principle of respect for persons finds expression in the regulations as a requirement for consent that requires that people, to the degree that they are capable, be given the opportunity to choose what shall or shall not happen to them. Consent is not just a form or a signature, but a process of information exchange that includes subject recruitment materials, verbal instructions, written materials, question/answer sessions and agreement documented by signature. The consent process can be analyzed as containing three components: information, comprehension and voluntariness.

> **Informed consent process:**
>
> - Information
>
> - Comprehension
>
> - Voluntariness

> Informed consent is a process or information exchange that takes place between the prospective subject and the investigator, before, during and sometimes after the study.

- *Information:* Most research codes and regulations establish specific items for disclosure. This is intended to ensure that research volunteers are given sufficient information. These items generally include: the research procedures, their purposes, risks and anticipated benefits, alternative procedures (especially where therapy is involved), and a statement offering the opportunity to ask questions and to withdraw at any time from the research.

> Freely given informed consent should be obtained from every volunteer before any research procedures have begun.

For judging how much and what sort of information should be provided, a standard of "the reasonable subject" should be used. This implies that the extent and nature of information provided should be such that a reasonable person has enough information to decide whether or not to participate in the research. Even when some direct benefit is anticipated, the subjects should understand clearly the range of risk and the voluntary nature of their participation.

In cases of research involving incomplete disclosure, research is justified only if it is clear that (1) incomplete disclosure is truly necessary to accomplish the goals of the research, (2) there are no undisclosed risks to subjects that are more than minimal, and (3) when appropriate, there is an adequate plan for debriefing subjects and for dissemination of research results to them. Information about risks should never be withheld for the purpose of eliciting the cooperation of subjects, and truthful answers should always be given to direct questions about the research. Care should be taken to distinguish cases in which disclosure would destroy or invalidate the research from cases in which disclosure would simply inconvenience the investigator or limit enrollment.

- *Comprehension:* The manner and context in which information is conveyed is as important as the information itself. For example, presenting information in a disorganized and rapid fashion, allowing too little time for consideration, or curtailing opportunities for questioning all may adversely affect a study subject's ability to make an informed choice. Because the subject's ability to understand is a function of intelligence, rationality, maturity and language, it is necessary to adapt the presentation of the information to the person's capabilities.

Investigators are responsible for ascertaining that the subject has comprehended the information. The investigator should encourage the person to ask questions. Investigators should make every attempt to ensure that the person understands the information, and they must give an opportunity to resolve any concerns before agreeing to participate in the study. Subjects should feel free to ask questions at any time – before, during and even after the experiment.

Special provision may need to be made when comprehension is severely limited — for example, by conditions of immaturity or mental disability. Even for these persons, however, respect requires giving them the opportunity to choose, to the extent they are able, whether or not to participate in research. In addition to this 'assent' process, respect for persons also requires seeking the permission of other parties in order to protect the subjects from harm.

- *Voluntariness:* An agreement to participate in research constitutes a valid consent only if voluntarily given. This condition of informed consent requires circumstances free of coercion and undue influence. Coercion occurs when a threat of harm is intentionally presented or implied by one person to another in order to obtain compliance. Undue influence, by contrast, occurs through an offer (implicit or explicit) of an excessive, unwarranted or improper reward (benefit) or other inappropriate assurances in order to obtain agreement. Investigators should assure that the circumstances (context) in which consent is obtained are free from undue influence. Subjects must understand that they are free to decline participation and to withdraw from the study at any time after it has begun.

2. Beneficence

Persons are treated in an ethical manner not only by respecting their decisions and protecting them from harm, but also by making efforts to secure their well being. Two general rules have been formulated as complementary expressions of beneficent actions: first, do not harm; and second, maximize possible benefits and minimize risks.

The obligations of beneficence affect both individuals and society. Effective ways of treating childhood diseases and promoting healthy development are benefits that serve to justify research, even when individual research subjects may not be direct beneficiaries. The principle of beneficence is reflected in regulations as a requirement to perform risk/benefit assessments.

Assessment of Risks and Benefits

The assessment of risks and benefits presents both an opportunity and a responsibility to gather systematic and comprehensive information about proposed research. For the investigator, it means examining whether the proposed research is properly designed. For a review committee, it is a requirement for determining whether the risks that will be presented to subjects are justified. For prospective volunteers, the assessment will assist their determination whether or not to participate.

The term "risk" refers to a possibility that harm may occur both in the chance (probability) of experiencing a harm and the severity (magnitude) of the envisioned harm. The term "benefit" is used in the research context to refer to something of positive value related to health or welfare. Accordingly, risk/benefit assessments are concerned with the probabilities and magnitudes of possible harms compared with anticipated benefits. While the most likely harms to research subjects are those of psychological or physical injury, other possible harms (e.g., social, legal and financial) should not be overlooked. Except for a narrow segment of research, the potential benefits accrue to society, and there are no benefits to individual study subjects. Often, determining the balance between personal risk borne by the study subject and potential societal benefit constitutes a key ethical dilemma in research ethics.

Risks and benefits of research may affect the individual subjects, the families of the subjects, and even society at large (or special groups within society). Beneficence requires both that we protect against risk of harm to study volunteers and also that we be concerned about the loss of the substantial benefits that might be gained from research.

The principle of beneficence is captured in risk/benefit assessments.

---

3. Justice

The principle of justice requires fairness in distribution. An injustice occurs when benefits to which a person is entitled are denied without good reason, or when burdens are imposed unduly. For example, the selection of research subjects should not systematically draw from certain classes (e.g., welfare patients, particular racial and ethnic minorities, or persons confined to institutions) simply because of their easy availability or their compromised position. Likewise, justice demands that research should not unduly involve persons from groups unlikely to be among the beneficiaries of subsequent applications of the research. This principle also requires inclusion of diverse populations/groups so that they may benefit from the findings of research. In the regulations, the principle of justice requires review of procedures for the selection of subjects and the outcome of those procedures.

Selection of Subjects

Justice is relevant to the selection of subjects of research at two levels: the individual and the social. Individual justice in the selection of subjects requires that researchers exhibit fairness. Justice requires fairness in the exclusion and inclusion criteria. Investigators and IRBs must consider subject selection issues including the encouragement by federal agencies for increasing enrollment of women, children and minorities. Social justice requires that distinction be drawn between classes of people asked to participate in any particular kind of research. Selection should be based upon the ability to bear burdens and on the appropriateness of placing further demands on already disadvantaged persons. Certain groups, such as the economically disadvantaged, the very sick and the institutionalized, given their dependent status and their frequently compromised capacity for free consent, should be protected against being involved in research solely for administrative convenience, or because they are easy to manipulate as a result of their illness and/or socioeconomic condition.

> The principle of justice is captured in the selection of research subjects.

Federal Regulations

Human Subject Protection Regulations

The federal regulations were directly derived from the ethical principles discussed above. In 1991, 17 federal departments and agencies adopted a common set of regulations, called 'the Common Rule,' governing human subject research sponsored by the federal government. The Common Rule was derived from the first of four subparts of the Department of Health and Human Services (DHHS) regulations for the protection of human subjects. These regulations date from 1981, when they were published together with Food and Drug Administration (FDA) human subject protection regulations as a response to the National Research Act of 1974 and the 1979 Belmont Report on research ethics. The Common Rule governs research that is conducted or supported by these federal agencies.

The equivalent FDA human subject protection regulations govern research with drugs, biologics and devices regardless of study sponsorship. The Common Rule has established three main protective mechanisms. They are: institutional assurances of compliance; review of research by an institutional review board (IRB); and requiring informed consent of subjects.

Protective Mechanisms Established by the Common Rule

1. Review of research by an IRB.

2. Informed consent of subjects.

3. Institutional assurances of compliance.

---

1. Review of Research by an Institutional Review Board (IRB)

Peer review and ethical review are key components of the research monitoring system. Scientific merit and methods are reviewed under a system of peer review at major research institutions. The purpose of the IRB is to review research and determine if the rights and welfare of human subjects involved in research are adequately protected. Institutions establish policies that ensure peer review and IRB review are properly conducted. By institutional policy, even studies that may otherwise be exempt from federal regulations may require review and/or verification of exempt status. Documents provided to peer review committees and IRBs by investigators must contain enough information to allow valid judgments about the science and ethics of the research.

The IRB has the authority to approve, require modification in (to approve), or disapprove all research activities, including proposed changes in previously approved human subject research. Based on factors including risk to subjects, IRBs determine which activities require continuing review more frequently than once a year and which need verification that no changes have occurred since previous review and approval.

- Before human subjects are involved in research, the IRB must consider:

  ⇨ The risks to the subjects.

  ⇨ The anticipated benefits to the subjects and others.

  ⇨ The importance of the knowledge that may reasonably result.

⇨ The informed consent process to be employed.

- The IRB must report promptly to the appropriate institutional officials, OPRR, FDA and any sponsoring agency of the federal government:

  ⇨ Any injuries to human subjects or other unanticipated problems involving risks to subjects or others.

  ⇨ Any serious or continuing noncompliance with regulations or requirements of the IRB.

  ⇨ Any suspension or termination of IRB approval for research.

- Initial and continuing review and approvals must be in compliance with federal regulations. Continuing reviews must be preceded by IRB receipt of appropriate progress reports from the investigator, including available study-wide findings.

- Research investigators must promptly report proposed changes in previously approved human subject research activities to the IRB. The proposed changes may not be initiated without IRB review and approval, except where necessary to eliminate apparent immediate hazards to the subjects.

2. Informed Consent of Subjects

As described in the Belmont Report, consent must be 1) informed, 2) understood and 3) voluntary. These are the hallmarks of consent and provide respect for persons by honoring their autonomy. The requirements to ensure 'legally effective' consent are intended to maximize the likelihood that consent is an informed autonomous decision.

Consent forms should reflect, in language that is understandable to volunteers, all relevant information about the study. Consent, whether written or oral, may not include waivers or the appearance of waivers of any of the person's legal rights. The same is true for releases (or appearance of releases) from liability for negligence of responsible parties. Technical language should be eliminated or explained in lay terms. Overly optimistic language should be avoided (e.g., "this product has been extensively and safely used elsewhere"). The form serves as a baseline of information for initial presentation and a reference source during the study as well as documentation of voluntary participation. Especially for long and/or complicated studies, investigators should stress to subjects the importance of keeping their copy of the consent form for reference. The original consent form, which is kept in the investigator's records, needs to be signed and dated by the subject.

3. Institutional Assurances of Compliance

Before a federal grant or contract can be awarded, the institution must file an 'Assurance of Compliance' with the government. This assurance may be valid for an individual grant (Single Project Assurance) or it may be valid for multiple grants (Multiple Project Assurances and Cooperative Project Assurances). In the Assurance, the institution agrees to apply the federal regulations, to monitor research, and to report instances of serious or continuing non-compliance. The Assurance also contains responsibilities of the investigator. Therefore, every investigator should read the Assurance and be familiar with its requirements.

> An Assurance imposes requirements on the institution and its researchers with respect to the conduct of human subject research.

The Office for Protection from Research Risk (OPRR) is the office within the federal government that negotiates Assurances for DHHS and oversees institutions' compliance with their Assurances. Research institutions must periodically reapply for and negotiate the terms of their Assurances as one mechanism by which the OPRR can address any concerns that may have come to its attention regarding the conduct of human subject research at a particular institution.

A Multiple Project Assurance (MPA) is only required for federally sponsored research, however, most MPA institutions voluntarily choose to extend the procedures and protections to all research conducted at the institution. MPA institutions must qualify for and maintain certain conditions and requirements in connection with the conduct and review of research projects. One fundamental condition of an Assurance is that the institution must establish and maintain an institutional review board (IRB) that oversees the conduct of research.

> The IRB review system is a requirement set forth in the Assurance.

MPA Violations

Given the potential ramifications of violating an Assurance, it is important for researchers to be compliant with the procedures established by the institution's Assurance for the review and approval of research , and to be compliant with applicable laws governing the conduct of human subject research.

If the OPRR determines that the obligations set forth in an Assurance have been violated, it has the authority to terminate or suspend the

Assurance. This means no federally-funded research can be conducted until the Assurance is reinstated. Typically the termination or suspension of an institution's Assurance arises in situations where there have been repeated and systematic violations of human subject research requirements by an institutional review board or by researchers, and as a result, the safety and welfare of research subjects is at risk.

Another significant sanction available to the OPRR is to temporarily suspend new enrollments in existing research protocols. The OPRR may also place certain restrictions on the institution's ability to conduct human subject research and/or require that the institution develop corrective actions. The OPRR would then monitor the implementation of these corrective actions by requiring the submission of periodic progress reports and possibly by conducting a site visit. If the institution failed to adequately apply the corrective actions, the more severe sanctions would be imposed.

Another restriction that has been utilized by the OPRR has been to remove a particular department or type of research from an institution's MPA. This requires all such research to obtain Single Project Assurances that are approved by the OPRR. This means the researchers, who are affected by this restriction, would have to send documents and other information to the OPRR for review, approval, and monitoring.

The OPRR also has the authority to impose sanctions on individual researchers. Included among the sanctions that may be imposed on an individual researcher are:

- Recommending to the DHHS that the researcher be barred from receiving federal funds for conducting research.

- Requiring OPPR approval for each study conducted by the researcher.

- Requiring the researcher undergo remedial training or education.

- Placing certain restrictions on the researcher's ability to conduct research (e.g. requiring supervision of the researcher).

Concerns regarding a particular researcher can come to the OPRR's attention through a number of mechanisms, including complaints by subjects. One mechanism is through a mandated IRB report to the OPRR. Federal regulations require the IRB to report to the OPRR (and the FDA as appropriate):

- Any serious or continuing non-compliance with regulations or requirements of the IRB.

- Any injuries or unanticipated problems involving research subjects.

- Any suspension or termination of IRB approval for research.

Violation of the obligations of Assurance can result in:

- Termination or suspension of the institution's Assurance.

- Suspension or restrictions to ongoing studies.

- Departmental restrictions.

- Individual restrictions.

Additional FDA Regulations and Sanctions

As stated previously, the FDA has regulations for the protection of human research subjects that are also based on the Belmont Report ethical principles. In addition, the FDA has specific regulations governing the way drugs, biologic products and medical devices may be used in clinical research settings. These regulations are also intended to protect subjects as well as to ensure sound data upon which to base approvals. Therefore, it is important that investigators who use FDA-regulated products be familiar with these regulations so that research is conducted in compliance. Like the other FDA regulations, these rules are contained in the Code of Federal Regulations (CFR) and are available in IRB and legal offices as well as on the Internet. The specific references for drugs and devices are 21 Parts 312, 314, 600, 812 and 814, all of which are included in the appendix.

The FDA works with individuals, companies and institutions to help promote compliance with the laws and regulations that govern clinical research. Most cases of noncompliance are due to misunderstanding of the regulations, or the responsibilities that individuals play in conducting clinical research. Institutions and individuals that work to resolve areas of noncompliance are generally met with the cooperation of the Agency. Disregard for the regulations and/or their intent, especially after initial goodwill efforts by the FDA, may lead to various levels of resistance or sanctions. Often correlated with the level to which research subjects are placed at risk, these include:

- Longer review of applications. Once a level of trust is broken with the FDA, additional safeguards, including more detailed review cycles, are often required.

- Warning Letters for specific documented concerns. These letters require immediate action, usually to cease all noncompliant activity until compliance is assured. Warning Letters are made public and posted on the

FDA Website and can be searched by individual, institution, company, date or compliance type. Frequently, although the Warning Letter may be specific to an individual investigator, it is directed to the institution and may result in action against the institution.

- Disqualification/debarment of individuals from clinical research (this can be temporary or permanent). The list of disqualified investigators is also posted on the FDA Website. Once a name is placed on the list, it stays even if the sanction is removed. It should be noted that this list is reviewed by companies as they choose investigators and sites for their clinical studies. It is also available for future employers, fellow investigators and researchers.

- Disqualification of institutions and/or IRBs from conducting or approving clinical research. Again, once an institution becomes known for noncompliance, it will take time and effort to re-establish trust with the agency.

- Other sanctions including seizures, injunctions, criminal charges and monetary penalties. These types of penalties are applied when there is evidence of willful serious disregard for the regulations and research subject safety. For individual researchers, these are often last resort efforts to halt criminal activity.

In addition to enacting regulations that implement the principles of the Belmont Report, the federal government has also enacted regulations governing misconduct in scientific research.

Scientific Misconduct

As a condition of accepting federal funding for research, institutions are required to adhere to the Public Health Service (PHS) regulations that apply to scientific misconduct. The regulations require that research institutions have written policies and procedures for investigating scientific misconduct. The current PHS definition of scientific misconduct is as follows:

Misconduct in science means fabrication, falsification, plagiarism or other practices that seriously deviate from those that are commonly accepted within the scientific community for proposing, conducting and reporting research. It does not include honest error or honest differences in interpretations or judgments of data.

The Public Health Service defines falsification to mean changing or falsifying existing data. It defines fabrication as the creation of data out of "thin air." It is important to note that honest errors or differences in interpretation are not considered misconduct. Although they are serious charges, incompetence and negligence are also not considered misconduct.

Within the definition of scientific misconduct, however, there is a significant gray area, particularly with respect to "other practices that seriously deviate from those that are commonly accepted." In light of this, if there is a concern that an individual may have engaged in practices that seriously deviate from acceptable research standards, the matter should be brought to the attention of the individual's immediate supervisor who can then further confer with the institutional officials regarding the appropriate action to be taken. If an individual has a concern with respect to his/her immediate supervisor, most institutions' policies designate other institutional officials who can be contacted.

> The definition of scientific misconduct does not include "honest errors" or "differences in interpretation of the data."

When an allegation regarding scientific misconduct is made, the regulations require that the institution investigate the allegation in two phases: the inquiry phase and the investigative phase. During the inquiry phase, the accused researcher, the complainant and anyone with knowledge that is relevant to the inquiry must be interviewed. The purpose of the inquiry phase is not to determine conclusively whether or not there was misconduct. Instead, the purpose of the inquiry phase is to determine whether or not there may be a basis to believe that misconduct could have occurred. PHS regulations require that the inquiry phase generally be completed within 60 days of receipt of the allegation. At the conclusion of the inquiry phase, the institution is required to write a report summarizing the results of the inquiry.

If, after the inquiry, institutional officials believe that misconduct may have occurred, the institution is required to conduct a more in-depth investigation. The institution is required to report its intention to conduct an investigation to the Office of Research Integrity. The Office of Research Integrity is a division of the PHS which oversees investigations of allegations of scientific misconduct.

> Institutions are required to report to the Office of Research Integrity when the institution decides to commence an in-depth investigation into an allegation of scientific misconduct.

When a further investigation is conducted into the allegation of misconduct (the investigative phase), the institution is required to interview the accused researcher, the complainant and others with knowledge relevant to the investigation. Relevant documents are also reviewed. At the conclusion of its investigation, the institution is required to write a report of its findings and its determination as to whether or not the individual accused of misconduct did commit scientific misconduct. The report is submitted to institutional officials, who determine the final action to be taken. The report is also submitted to the Office of Research Integrity, which has the authority to either accept or reject the findings. In general, the investigative phase takes no more than 120 days. The PHS regulations require that inquiries and investigations into allegations of misconduct be conducted in as confidential a manner as possible without compromising the ability to conduct an effective investigation.

Individuals who have in good faith made an allegation of misconduct ("whistle-blowers") should not be the object of retaliation. Indeed, retaliation against a whistle-blower who made an allegation of misconduct in good faith, may itself, be construed as an act of misconduct.

> Retaliation against a "whistle-blower" may be construed as an act of misconduct.

If an individual is found guilty of scientific misconduct, there is a range of penalties that the institution and the Office of Research Integrity may utilize. With respect to the institution, penalties may range from requiring further training for the individual or supervision to terminating his or her appointment. The Office of Research Integrity may impose penalties that range from researcher supervision to the maximal penalty of researcher debarment from conducting federally-funded research. Additionally, in some instances, the institution or Office of Research Integrity may require that any publication related to the research in question be retracted or corrected.

CHAPTER 3

ROLES AND RESPONSIBILITIES OF INSTITUTIONS IN HUMAN SUBJECT RESEARCH

Objectives

At the conclusion of this chapter, readers will be able to:

- Describe the responsibilities of research institutions and federal regulatory agencies in conducting clinical research.

- Discuss the legal basis and the intent of the regulations governing clinical research.

- Describe the term "Good Clinical Practice" and how it applies to clinical research.

Introduction

The roles and responsibilities of the federal agencies, institutions and investigators in conducting human subject research are defined in federal and state laws and regulations. This chapter provides a general review of the institution, IRBs and federal agencies roles.

Research Institution

The research institution bears responsibility for compliance with the Department of Health and Human Services (DHHS) and Food and Drug Administration (FDA) regulations for the performance of all research activities that involve human subjects. Institutions are required to install additional safeguards for research in vulnerable populations. This is true for research conducted at sites that are under the direction of any employee or agent of the institution. The institution has responsibility for educating researchers on issues of scientific integrity as well as the mandated responsibility to investigate cases of scientific misconduct. In addition, the institution has a responsibility to enforce a policy on conflict of interest.

Issues That Require Institutional Review

- Ethical (i.e., IRB) Review (of the protocol and informed consent).

- Administrative Review of Proposals, Contracts and Grants.

- Scientific Peer Review.

1. Ethical Review

Institutions ensure the protection of the rights, safety and welfare of all research subjects by assuring that an IRB operating in compliance with federal regulations is in place. By regulation, when approving research, the IRB must determine that the following requirements are satisfied:

- Risks to subjects are minimized:

  ⇨ by using procedures that are consistent with sound research design and that do not unnecessarily expose subjects to risk, and

  ⇨ whenever appropriate, by using procedures already being performed on the subjects for diagnostic or treatment purposes.

- Risks are reasonable in relation to anticipated benefits to subjects, if any, and to the importance of the expected knowledge. In evaluating risks and benefits, the IRB considers only those risks and benefits that may result directly from the research (as distinguished from risks and benefits that people would have even if not participating in the research).

- Selection of subjects is equitable. In making this assessment, the IRB takes into account the purpose(s) of the research and the setting in which the research will be conducted.

- Informed consent will be sought from each prospective subject, or the subject's legally authorized representative unless waived in accordance with regulations.

- Informed consent will be appropriately documented, usually with a signed written consent form.

- Where appropriate, the research plan makes provisions for monitoring the data collected to ensure the safety of subjects.

- Where appropriate, there are provisions to protect the privacy of participants and to maintain the confidentiality of data.

- Additional safeguards are included in the study to protect the rights and welfare of subjects when some or all of themare likely to be vulnerable to coercion or undue influence (children, prisoners, pregnant women, handicapped, mentally disabled persons or economically or educationally disadvantaged persons).

The IRB reviews the investigator's study design/protocol for the information it needs to make the above determinations. IRBs grant approval based upon the information provided and expect the researcher to abide by the protocol as written. Any changes in the study must receive prior approval by the IRB before being instituted. Industry sponsors may require that any changes made by the IRB be relayed to them for concurrence.

Some funding/sponsoring organizations require IRB review of projects before they can be considered for funding/sponsoring. Often, the funding/sponsoring organization's review results in changes to the study design. It is essential that the investigator know that, if the study is to be funded and conducted, all changes must be reviewed and approved by the IRB before the study may begin.

> To ensure an effective review by the IRB, the board must be provided with certain critical information, including: the protocol/study design, consent form(s) and subject recruiting materials.

This is also true for changes required by a regulatory agency. For example, in the Investigational New Drug Application (IND)/Investigational Device Exemption (IDE) review process, if the FDA requires changes to the study, these changes must be submitted to the IRB for approval. Changes are submitted to the IRB as amendments.

After the initial approval, all studies must undergo continuing review by the IRB to ensure that: 1) the risk-benefit relationship of the research remains acceptable, 2) the informed consent process and documents are still appropriate, and 3) the enrollment of subjects has been equitable. By federal regulation, the maximum period between these IRB reviews is one year. As part of the continuing review, the IRB will assess appropriate information such as enrollment figures and demographics; adverse events and unanticipated problems; subject withdrawals; preliminary study results and publications and the consent process. The investigator is responsible for applying for continuing review in a timely manner to ensure IRB approval is continuous. If a study is not re-approved before the study's expiration date, it is automatically suspended until formal notice of re-approval from the IRB is received. Sponsors require notification of IRB approvals (initial and continuing).

2. Administrative Review of Proposals, Contracts and Grants

Most research organizations establish a sponsored-programs office that reviews and authorizes proposals to external sponsors, accepts grants and reviews or approves contracts for all associated researchers.

This office generally ensures that proposals and associated budgets are in compliance with institution and sponsor policies (including IRB review where appropriate) and that investigator assurances are current. These assurances include a determination that a financial interest does not have a significant effect upon the design, conduct or reporting of the proposed study. Generally, if the investigator has a financial interest in the sponsor funding the clinical study, the institution will need to make a determination if the conflict can be managed. Some institutions will not accept funding if this situation exists.

By authorizing a proposal to an external sponsor, the institution is:

- Stating that in the institution's best estimation, the statement of work or protocol can be performed at the proposed funding level.

- Any unique policies of the institution have been considered.

- The proposal meets the requirements of the potential sponsor.

- The institution will comply with all federal and state laws and regulations, as well as institutional policies.

This office addresses contractual issues inherent in clinical research contracts, such as ownership of data, appropriate sharing of liability, responsibility for subject injury and the protection of publication rights for researchers. This office is also responsible for negotiating terms on which sponsor confidential information will be accepted.

Institutional review and administration does not negate the responsibility of the investigator.

3. Scientific Peer Review

Peer review ensures that sound research design and methods are employed. Institutional peer review committees focus on the scientific concerns of studies. The composition and qualifications of the research team are generally examined and they may also consider resource issues.

Federal Agencies

While several federal agencies, such as Department of Education, Department of Defense and the National Science Foundation, fund and regulate research, they generally follow the lead of the Department of Health and Human Services (DHHS).

Department of Health and Human Services (DHHS)

Besides the FDA (discussed separately below), the DHHS houses several other agencies that regulate or fund research. The National Institutes of Health's (NIH) mission is to uncover new knowledge that leads to better public health. The NIH's role in research is primarily to conduct studies with its own investigators and to provide funding for research projects at other institutions, especially multi-site national studies. To a lesser extent, other DHHS agencies also function in the role of research conductor/sponsor. Examples include the Center for Disease Control and Prevention (CDC) and the Agency for Health Care Policy and Research (AHCPR).

While the funding agencies within the DHHS are not regulatory, they are responsible for promulgating regulations applicable to Public Health Service (PHS) funded research. An example is the conflict of interest rule that establishes standards and procedures to be followed by institutions to ensure that the design, conduct or reporting of research funded under PHS grants, cooperative agreements or contracts will not be biased by any conflicting financial interest of its investigators.

The Office for the Protection from Research Risk (OPRR) regulates, in a manner similar to FDA, research in human subjects for studies conducted with DHHS funds in order to protect the rights and safety of subjects. This includes regulations for the institutional review of protocols and informed consent documents.

The Office of Research Integrity (ORI) conducts investigations regarding misconduct in research. As a condition of accepting federal funding for research, institutions are required to adhere to the Public Health Service (PHS) regulations that apply to scientific misconduct. If an individual is found guilty of scientific misconduct, there is a range of penalties that the institution and the ORI may impose.

> The Office of Research Integrity (ORI) conducts investigations regarding misconduct in research.

Food and Drug Administration (FDA)

The Food and Drug Administration (FDA) is the federal consumer protection agency within the Department of Health and Human Services (DHHS) that enforces the Food, Drug and Cosmetic Act (the FD&C Act) and related federal public health laws. According to these laws, only drugs, biologics and medical devices that have been proven safe and effective can be marketed.

To allow for research to determine the safety and effectiveness of new (i.e., investigational) drugs, biologics or device products, the FDA has established regulations that govern study sponsors, investigators and institutional review boards.

Prior to the initiation of a research study with an investigational product, an application to FDA for exemption from the FD&C Act is usually required.

> Although FDA oversight may not be necessary, the protocol and informed consent still needs to undergo review by the IRB.

The FDA monitors research through review of required reports from investigators, sponsors, institutions and IRBs as well as through a program of on-site inspections and audits. The Biomedical Monitoring Program inspects all the players in the research enterprise.

Good Clinical Practice (GCP)

In the United States, GCPs have been based primarily upon FDA policy and regulation. In the last few years, however, a movement toward international GCP standards has occurred. The International Conference on Harmonization (ICH) is composed of expert working groups from various regulatory bodies in the European Union, Japan and the United States. ICH published a guideline for Good Clinical Practice (GCP). This worldwide GCP document offers standardization for clinical trials.

Good Clinical Practice (GCP) is an ethical and scientific quality standard for designing, conducting, monitoring, recording, auditing, analyzing and reporting trials that involve participation of human subjects. GCPs are consistent with ethical principles put forth in the Declaration of Helsinki. The main purposes of GCP are:

1. To protect human subjects during clinical studies, and

2. To protect patients who might receive approved products in the future.

FDA and ICH regulations are the basis for good clinical practices that govern clinical research. Compliance with this standard provides public assurance that the rights, safety and well-being of trial subjects are protected, and that the clinical trial data are credible and accurate.

> GCPs offer protection for human subjects in clinical trials.

There is no one source of guidance for GCPs. They are embodied within laws, regulations and guidelines such as:

- Ethical codes
- IRB and consent regulations.
- Guidelines on the obligations of investigators, sponsors and monitors.
- Code of Federal Regulations pertaining to drugs and devices.
- Form FDA 1572.
- ICH Guidelines.
- Official guidance documents.

> Following GCPs ensures the accuracy and reliability of data generated in the course of a clinical trial.

Compliance with GCPs during clinical trials will ensure that:

- The rights and safety of human subjects are not compromised.
- Appropriately and adequately trained staff manage the study.
- The study is carefully documented.
- Protocol is strictly adhered to.

> GCPs are recognized as the standard operating procedures
> of a clinical trial.

GCPs, therefore, encompass all aspects of a clinical trial including (but not limited to):

- Obtaining informed consent.

- Documenting accurate case histories.

- Maintaining complete "paper trails" for all study documents.

- Reporting adverse events.

- Proper record retention.

CHAPTER 4

THE ROLES AND RESPONSIBILITIES OF THE INVESTIGATOR AND THE STUDY PROCESS

> ### Objectives:
>
> At the conclusion of this chapter, readers will be able to:
>
> - Describe the roles and responsibilities of the investigator and research team.
>
> - List the items that should be included in a protocol (study design).
>
> - List the required elements of a consent form.
>
> - Describe the issues to consider in subject recruitment for a study.

Introduction

The complex responsibilities of conducting research can make the investigator's role difficult and challenging. On the other hand, once the investigator understands the responsibilities involved, research can be rewarding for both the investigator and for the subjects who participate. The study process begins before the first subject is entered, and continues after the last subject has completed the study. This chapter provides an overview of the roles of the research team members, the responsibilities of investigators, and the steps involved in the process of conducting a successful research study.

Investigator's Role and Responsibilities

Investigators share with IRBs and sponsors the responsibility for ensuring that study subjects are adequately protected. They are required to assure that the IRB reviewing the study is in compliance with federal regulations. Studies must be properly designed so that they are scientifically sound and likely to yield valid results. Investigators must be appropriately qualified to conduct the research. The investigator is responsible for ensuring that the research is conducted according to the research design as approved by the IRB. Respect for study subjects' rights and dignity requires that informed consent be obtained before a person participates in a study.

> The safety and welfare of research subjects ultimately rests with the investigator.

Professional Judgment

The ultimate responsibility for the acceptable conduct of research with human subjects rests with the investigator. Only sound professional judgment can ensure the protection of study subjects. It is up to the investigator to see that:

- The personal dignity and autonomy of the research volunteer are respected.

- Subjects are protected from harm by maximizing anticipated benefits and minimizing possible risks.

- The benefits and burdens of research are shared fairly.

The challenge arises in deciding how to protect the study subjects while also achieving progress in science. Although the two objectives are not mutually exclusive, they also are not without conflict. Understanding the distinction between research and practice is fundamental to resolving any conflict that may arise. It is also essential to recognize the potential for confusion on the part of the subject (e.g., patient, client, student) about his/her relationship to the investigator, who may also be his/her physician, social worker or educator.

The purpose of medical or behavioral practice is to provide diagnosis, preventative treatment or therapy. "Practice" involves interventions designed solely to enhance the well-being of the patient or client. These interventions are undertaken because there is a reasonable expectation of a successful outcome. "Research" constitutes activities designed to contribute to generalizable knowledge. Typically, a set of activities is consistently applied to groups of individuals in order to test a hypothesis and draw conclusions. The activities are not necessarily therapeutic in nature.

The line between practice and research is often blurred. Experimental procedures do not necessarily constitute research and often, research and practice occur simultaneously. The investigator's professional judgment is essential to maintain the integrity of the research process and to keep the study volunteer informed of his/her role in the process and relationship with the investigator(s). People who are used as research subjects without their consent may be wronged, even if they are not harmed.

> Professional judgment is required throughout the research process to provide the necessary checks and balances.

Professional judgment is required throughout the research process to provide the necessary checks and balances. No balance of research/therapy is acceptable if it is likely to result in less than adequate care for the subject. It can be tempting to value knowledge more highly than basic human rights when excited by the prospect of a new methodology or new understanding of biological processes. To avoid this, consider the following questions before undertaking a new study.

- What types of people will be enrolled? Address this from an ethical perspective as well as on the basis of entry criteria.

    ⇨ What are their alternatives?

    ⇨ Would some potential subjects incur more risks than others? Accrue more benefits?

    ⇨ Are all subjects capable of understanding the consent process?

- What is your relationship to the subject?

    ⇨ Are you also their care-giver?

    ⇨ Do they delegate their decisions for participating in a protocol to you?

    ⇨ Are they comfortable asking you questions?

- How do you treat someone with an intervention that has not been proven to be safe or effective?

- Are you so involved with the "science," publishing, presenting or grant review, that there is significant potential for conflict?

These are among the many questions that investigators must ask themselves regularly.

There is no standard operating procedure to address the potential issues that can arise when human subjects are used for research. Because the future of science depends on the good will and trust of the public, investigators must understand and meet their duty to human subjects.

Study Conduct

The investigator is personally responsible for the conduct of the research project and for the actions of personnel under his/her supervision. Many studies are conducted by one investigator, commonly referred to as the principal investigator (PI) or clinical investigator (CI).

The investigator of a study is required by law to conduct the study according to the:

- Investigational plan (including the protocol and IRB stipulations).

- Institutional policies.

- All applicable regulations.

Additional responsibilities for FDA-regulated studies are to:

- Comply with the signed investigators' statement (Form FDA 1572).

- Supervise use of the test article(s).

- Maintain accurate study records.

- Maintain control of all test articles, ensuring that no people other than those identified to the FDA are given access to the test article.

> The investigator is responsible for the study conduct.

The term 'co-principal-investigator' (co-PI) is used when a study is conducted by more than one investigator, each of whom assumes equal responsibility for the conduct of the study and adherence to the regulations. The reasons for a study being conducted by co-principal-investigators are varied. For example, co-PIs are often used in drug studies when an investigator has multiple sites where different investigators are responsible at each location.

Principal investigators, and co-investigators, must be qualified by education, training and experience to assume responsibility for the proper conduct of the research project. They should meet all the qualifications specified by the applicable regulatory requirements and provide evidence of such qualifications through an up-to-date *curriculum vitae* and relevant documentation as requested by the sponsor, the IRB and/or regulatory authorities.

Administration of the Study

Because investigators are required to conduct the study in accordance with institutional policies and all applicable regulations, their responsibilities go beyond the scientific and clinical conduct of the study itself.

Other responsibilities of investigators include:

- Compliance with federal/state laws and regulations, including a conflict of interest disclosure.

- Assuming fiscal management.

- Supervising and training of students, postdocs and residents.

- Complying with the terms and conditions of the sponsor's award, for example, non-disclosure of sponsor confidential information.

- Submission of all technical, progress, invention and financial reports on a timely basis.

By accepting the study, the investigator must remain cognizant of these responsibilities. Violations or delinquencies may result in loss of funding or even debarment in certain instances.

Research Team Role and Responsibilities

The composition of the research team may vary according to the scope and complexity of the research project and the number of investigational sites involved. In some instances the study may be conducted by one individual. Most biomedical studies involve the expertise of a team of individuals.

When the investigator delegates responsibility to various members of his/her research team (e.g., survey instruments, follow-up tests, exams, procedures performed by others), the investigator must maintain a good working relationship with all team members to ensure they perform these procedures as the protocol requires. It is recommended that the research team meet periodically to discuss study progress and problems as they arise. It may be helpful to keep notes or minutes, thereby documenting that the investigator is effectively managing the study.

Subinvestigator

A subinvestigator is any team member (e.g., junior faculty, graduate student, resident, lab staff) other than an investigator, who may help in the design and conduct of the investigation, but does not actually direct its conduct. Put another way, the subinvestigator can be any member of a research team designated and supervised by the investigator to perform study-related procedures and/or to make important study-related decisions. The investigator often delegates responsibility to others within their sphere of control. Any one of these individuals could be considered a subinvestigator.

Subinvestigators designated and supervised by the investigator should be qualified by education, professional qualifications and experience to perform the procedures delegated by the principal investigator. Typically, the competency of a subinvestigator can usually be documented with a *curriculum vitae*.

> The subinvestigator may help conduct the study, but
> does not direct it.

Clinical Research Coordinator (CRC) or Study Coordinator

The Clinical Research Coordinator (CRC) is a research professional working for and under the direction of an investigator. The CRC is responsible for screening and recruiting subjects, collecting and recording clinical data and maintaining clinical supplies where applicable.

Other Team Members

The principal investigator can delegate study specific tasks, but the level of responsibility must coincide with the experience and/or capabilities of the team member. Other team members may include a variety of professionals, statisticians, laboratory technicians and administrative staff.

The investigator should always document in writing the responsibilities delegated to all members of the research team. The time period that each team member participated should also be documented. This is important in the event team members change during the course of the study.

Study Process

The study process includes protocol development, departmental scientific review, funding applications, administrative review of contract/grants and the application to the IRB. When an investigator is developing a study design, it may be useful to consult with the IRB regarding human subject protections. Other institution officials and administrators should be advised and consulted as necessary. When an award is made, most institutional and sponsor policies require that the protocol and associated contract be formally accepted by the investigator and an official of the institution.

Protocol (Study Design) Development

The protocol is a formal document that establishes the conditions under which the research is to be conducted. When writing the protocol, the investigator should include applicable sections – example items are listed below:

- The specific scientific objectives (aims of the research).

- Budget, personnel and facility considerations.

- The research method(s) and all procedures.

- The statistical/analytical methods to be used, including justification for the number of subjects expected to participate.

- If a data monitoring committee is used, describe its operation (e.g., membership, stopping rules and frequency of review).

- Security measures to protect the research data.

- Human subject issues such as:

  ⇨ The inclusion criteria.

  ⇨ The exclusion criteria.

  ⇨ Justification for any inclusion of vulnerable subjects (e.g., those with limited autonomy or those in subordinate positions).

  ⇨ The intended gender distribution of the subjects. [Note: Women of childbearing potential may not be routinely excluded from participating in research.]

  ⇨ The age range of the subjects. [Note: Special considerations apply to NIH funded research, which must address the inclusion of children.]

  ⇨ The intended racial and ethnic distribution of the subjects.

  ⇨ The potential risks associated with the study.

  ⇨ Any potential benefit(s).

  ⇨ Alternatives that are available should the subject select not to participate in the study.

⇨ The recruitment methods.

⇨ Who will obtain consent and how the process of informed consent will be structured.

⇨ If all subjects will not be capable of giving consent, describe additional protections.

⇨ Assessment of understanding of the information presented.

⇨ Justification of any non-disclosure and description of post-study debriefing.

⇨ Justification of any costs that the subjects will incur.

⇨ Description of any reimbursements or incentives such as cash payments.

Informed Consent Requirements

The regulations, codes and institutional policies state items that must be disclosed to satisfy the 'informed' consent requirement. Although each research study involving human subjects is unique, federal regulations require that all consent forms contain the following information elements:

• Introduction (with statement that this is research).

• Purpose of study.

• Description of study procedures (identifying any that are experimental).

• Duration of subject involvement.

• Potential risks or discomforts of participation.

• Potential benefits of participation.

• Alternatives (medical treatments or other courses of action, if any).

• Confidentiality of records statement.

• Compensation for injury statement (for greater than minimal risk studies).

• Contact persons.

• Statement of voluntary participation.

It is important to include several other elements of information if they apply to the study and are important for subjects to know. These include:

• Unforeseen risks statement (if applicable).

- Reasons for involuntary termination of participation (if applicable).

- Additional costs to participate (if any).

- Consequences for withdrawal (adverse health/welfare effects if any).

- New findings statement (to be provided if relevant).

- Number of subjects (if it may have an impact on the decision to participate).

- Payments (incentives and/or expense reimbursements if any).

Informed consent is not just a form or a signature, but a process of information exchange that includes:

- subject recruitment materials.

- verbal instructions.

- written materials.

- question/answer sessions.

- agreement documented by signature.

Recruitment Issues

Recruiting subjects is one of the most important, and sometimes difficult and time-consuming, aspects of conducting research. Recruiting is an aspect of a study that must be considered before the study and must continue throughout the duration of the trial.

The investigator should determine feasibility of recruiting subjects prior to accepting a study.

Recruitment issues to consider before conducting a study:

- Competing studies.

    ⇨ *Other studies being conducted that require same population, and may deplete availability of potential subjects.*

- Time frames.

    ⇨ *The anticipated start/stop dates of the study period may change. This may affect subject availability, investigator workload, etc.*

- Subject availability.

  ⇨ *The protocol inclusion/exclusion criteria define the population to be studied. The characteristics of the subject population are a major consideration in recruitment.*

  ⇨ *The feasibility of recruiting this subject population must be determined prior to accepting the study.*

- Recruitment strategy.

  ⇨ *The recruiting methods that will be used will affect the numbers and mix of potential subjects.*

- Gender of the subjects.

  ⇨ *Equitable inclusion of both men and women in research is important to ensure that each receives an equal share of the benefits and neither carries a disproportionate burden. Therefore, subjects of both genders should be included unless there are medical and/or scientific contraindications. [Note: Women of childbearing potential should not be routinely excluded from participating in clinical research].*

- Age range of subjects.

  ⇨ *Participation of adult subjects in research should not be age-restricted unless there is scientific and/or medical justification.*

  ⇨ *Participation of children should be considered unless there is sound scientific or medical justification for exclusion.*

- Racial and ethnic origin.

  ⇨ *Within the limitations imposed by the population of the study site(s), research should include sufficient enrollment of persons of diverse racial/ethnic backgrounds in order to ensure that the benefits and burdens of research participation are distributed in an equitable manner.*

> Women of childbearing potential may not be routinely excluded from participating in research.

A variety of recruitment methods and materials are used by researchers, including:

- Formal referrals or informal word-of-mouth.

- Health workshops, screenings and health fairs.

- Internet.

- Direct advertising.

- Community meeting places (barber shops, recreation spots, etc.).

- Computerized database.

- Chart/record review.

It is unacceptable to use confidential/private data to which the investigator would not ordinarily have access to approach subjects for a research study (i.e., cold contacting). The initial contact with potential subjects should be made by those having legitimate access to the information. This person would convey referral or contact information.

Direct advertising is a frequently used recruitment technique. Direct advertising is recruitment information intended for the prospective subjects. Direct advertising types include flyers, posters, newspaper ads and press releases. Television and radio spots, websites and electronic mailers are also considered direct advertisements. All direct advertising must have IRB approval before being used for recruiting subjects. It is considered part of the informed consent and subject selection process. In this regard, all direct advertising must:

- Be reviewed by the IRB for the information contained and the mode of communication.

- Not state or imply a certainty of favorable outcome or other benefits beyond what is outlined in the consent document and protocol.

- Not be coercive or use undue pressures.

- Not be misleading to subjects.

Advertising don'ts:

- No misleading text.

- No claims of safety, efficacy, equivalence or superiority.

- No overemphasis of payment.

- No overstatement of benefits.

Advertising for recruitment into investigational drug, biologic or device studies should not use terms such as "new treatment," "new medication" or "new drug" because it inappropriately implies that safety and effectiveness have been determined.

Advertising to recruit subjects should generally be limited to:

- The name and address of the investigator and/or research facility.

- The purpose of study or condition under study.

- A brief description of eligibility requirements.

- Benefits of participation.

- Time commitment required of participants.

- Whom to contact for more information.

Advertising pointers:

- Avoid acronyms. They may not be understood by the target audience.

- Place the ad carefully to reach the appropriate audience.

- Advertise frequently in the right places.

- Measure the effectiveness of the advertising technique. Modify tactics as needed.

Payment to Subjects for Participation

Payment for participation requires conscientious judgment calls on the part of the researchers and the IRB. It is not uncommon for people to be paid for their participation in research, especially for research with no direct benefit to the subjects, for example, survey completion or the early phases of investigational drug, biologic or device development.

The amount of payment must not be an undue inducement of the person to participate in the research. Frequently study subjects are reimbursed an amount to cover transportation, parking, lunch, etc. — costs associated with participation. The amount of payment and payment schedule should be presented to the IRB. Information regarding payments (including amounts and scheduling of payments) must be included in the consent form. A prorated payment system should be used. This means that payments are earned/given as the study progresses, and that subjects do not have to complete the entire study to be paid. A reasonable bonus for completion of a study may be paid if it does not unduly influence participants to continue when they would have withdrawn otherwise. How the payment is prorated should be specified.

The payments to subjects for participation is not considered a benefit, it is a recruitment incentive.

> **Prorated system of subject payment means:**
>
> - Payments are earned as the study progresses.
>
> - Participants do not have to complete the entire study to be paid.

Protocol Adherence

The investigator must follow the protocol. This is a specific requirement for the investigator's compliance with the regulations. The time to evaluate study procedures and for the inclusion/exclusion criteria is while the protocol is in its draft form. Once deemed 'final,' it is a violation of the protocol to not comply with the established procedures and inclusion/exclusion criteria. [Note: Sponsors may provide the investigator with only a final protocol. The investigator must decide in advance if he/she can comply with the entire document **as written**. There may be no opportunity for protocol input].

All amendments must be approved by the IRB and sponsor (if applicable) prior to their implementation. Any deviations from the protocol should be documented and for sponsored studies, the sponsor should be consulted in advance if a deviation is requested. Most industrial sponsors will call unauthorized deviations protocol violations and will not be willing to pay for these data.

EXCEPTION: The investigator may deviate from the protocol to eliminate an immediate hazard to subjects, without prior IRB approval. This deviation from the protocol, along with the rationale, is considered a protocol amendment. The IRB should be notified as soon as possible regarding such a change.

While most common in drug and medical device studies, adverse events could occur to human subjects in almost any research study. Investigators have the responsibility to monitor research subjects to detect difficulties, discomfort and other more severe reactions. When these are encountered, the investigator should take appropriate steps to remedy the immediate situation as well as minimize the chance for recurrences. Adverse events must be reported to the IRB. If they were expected and listed in the consent form, they can usually be reported at the time of continuing review. If they are unexpected, especially if severe, adverse events should be reported when they occur to the IRB for review. IRBs have defined time limits for adverse event reporting by investigators.

If changes to the research design and/or the consent form are to be made, they must be approved by the IRB before they are implemented. Changes in the consent form, particularly when new risks are added, may require re-consent of currently enrolled subjects if the IRB deems it necessary. Re-consent is documented in study records or through the use of a consent addendum or new consent form.

> The investigator (or designee) should document and explain all deviations from the protocol.

Investigators on industry-sponsored studies should also be aware that there also may be special circumstances (e.g., open label therapeutic use) when the sponsor may allow a person into a clinical trial who does not meet the protocol's inclusion/exclusion criteria. This must FIRST be approved by the sponsor and documented in the study records.

Some studies, such as industry-sponsored drug trials and cooperative group studies, include routine auditing or monitoring. The study monitor reviews adherence to the protocol at the monitoring visits. Reviews include, but are not limited to:

- Review of subject eligibility criteria to verify that no inclusion/exclusion violations occur.

- Scheduling of subject visits and review of subject compliance for visits

- Evaluation procedures.

- Follow-up of study drop outs.

- Records of disposition and use of investigational agent.

- Thoroughness of source documentation.

- Accuracy of case report forms as compared to source documentation.

> Discovery of major or repeated noncompliance with the protocol can result in termination of the investigator's participation in a trial, or even disqualification as an investigator.

Enrollment Incentive Payments to Researchers

Incentives include payments from study sponsors (or their contract research organizations) to research institutions/individuals for purposes of increasing the numbers and/or rate of enrollment of people into research studies. Incentives not only include monetary payments, but may also include reimbursements for travel or other expenses that may or may not be related to the study. There are legal and ethical issues associated with incentives.

Incentive categories include:

- Finder's Fees: payment to physicians (or others) for referring subjects to investigators.

- Bonus Payments: payment to the investigator, study coordinators, enrollers or the institution for enhanced enrollment (these are not associated with actual costs).

- Additional Cost Payments: payment that is based upon additional costs of enrollment that were not originally anticipated.

Generally, finder's fees and bonus payments to encourage recruitment of subjects are not acceptable. These payments may compromise the integrity of studies or may give an appearance of affecting the judgment of the investigator/research team. In some cases, such payments may violate regulations and institutional policies.

Additional per-subject payment for increased costs associated with enhanced and/or accelerated enrollment or additional procedures required by the sponsor is usually acceptable. All incentive payment agreements should be reviewed by appropriate institutional offices, even if they are introduced after the clinical trial agreement is executed. This review is intended to ensure that the consent language is uniform, that incentives are appropriate and that incentives are uniformly applied to all enrolled subjects.

CHAPTER 5

FDA-REGULATED RESEARCH ISSUES

Objectives

At the conclusion of this chapter, readers will be able to:

- Describe the Food and Drug Administration (FDA) regulations as they apply to drugs/biologics and medical devices.

- Discuss the responsibilities of the sponsor in FDA-regulated research.

- Describe the study process for industry-sponsored studies.

- Discuss sponsor – investigator – institution interactions.

- Identify the responsibilities of the investigator who assumes the additional role of the sponsor.

Introduction

The FDA regulates drugs, biologics and devices used in the diagnosis, cure, mitigation, treatment or prevention of disease in man and animals. This section addresses FDA-regulated clinical research and the responsibilities of industry sponsors, the additional study processes that industry sponsors may require and the additional responsibilities that investigators take on when they chose to sponsor a study with an FDA-regulated drug, biologic or device.

The FDA conducts a thorough review of drugs, biologics and medical devices for safety and effectiveness for a given indication prior to granting approval for marketing. Before release to the marketplace, the FDA and the sponsor write the package insert (also referred to as the "labeling"). This document summarizes what the FDA has determined to be the safe and effective use of the product. The FDA then exempts further clinical studies that are conducted according to this labeling from the IND regulations. The FDA does not, however, exempt such studies from the human subjects protection regulations. All research studies with FDA-regulated products that involve human subjects are required to undergo review by an IRB, even if exempt from IND/IDE filing.

> Exemption from IND/IDE regulations is NOT an exemption from IRB review.

Drugs and Biologics/INDs

If the subject population is different than that indicated in the labeling, it becomes a clinical judgment and/or ethical question as to whether this new population is at greater risk of injury with the product than the indicated population. The use of a placebo for blinding a study does not, by itself, require the filing of an IND. Examples of when an IND is warranted because of greater risk include:

• Increased dose.

• Different route of administration.

• Longer duration.

• If the research population is "vulnerable."

• If there is reason to believe that this population has different pharmacokinetic or pharmacodynamic responses from the indicated population.

> Exemptions to the IND process apply as long as the product is used according to the product labeling (dose, duration, patient population, etc.).

Research involving a drug or biologic that has not yet reached the marketplace requires an IND. The FDA carefully and critically reviews these applications and will only allow human exposure if they feel that the risks of the exposure are reasonable. The IND application usually contains evidence of safety and tolerability in animals, a controlled method of manufacture with assurances of the identity of the final drug product, specific tests for significant toxins or toxic ingredients and a well developed clinical plan that minimizes the risks for human subjects.

Form FDA 1572

Each investigator participating in drug or biologic studies, subject to the IND regulations, is required to sign the Form FDA 1572. By signing the 1572, also referred to as the "statement of investigator," the investigator agrees to conduct the investigation according to the provisions listed on the Form. The back of Form FDA 1572 lists the commitments the investigator is making to the FDA for conduct of the study.

The Form FDA 1572 is often referred to as the "hanging paper" because it is a criminal offense to sign the document if it contains false information or if commitments made within the signed document are ignored. These investigator commitments should be reviewed prior to signing this form. Investigators have been prosecuted based on this signature in the past.

The FDA Form 1572 requires the names of the individuals involved in the clinical research project.

Investigator: The name and address of the investigator is required. If there are co-principal-investigators involved in the project, the co-PIs' names and addresses can be presented in one of two ways: 1) both co-investigators' names are entered and each signs the one form or 2) each co-investigator completes and signs a separate form. The person/persons signing as the investigator assumes full responsibility for the proper conduct of the study.

Subinvestigator: The form also requests the "Names of the subinvestigators (e.g., research fellows, residents, associates) who will be assisting the investigator in the conduct of the investigation(s)." The issue of who should be listed as a subinvestigator frequently causes confusion for investigators. The regulations are not specific regarding this issue. Normally, those individuals should be listed who perform significant trial-related procedures and/or make study-related medical decisions regarding the diagnosis and treatment of the condition under investigation, e.g., physicians, hospital residents, specialists.

It is the research sponsor who submits the completed, signed Form FDA 1572 to the FDA. A sponsor may request that everyone associated with the research project be listed on the form. Different sponsors have different requirements, thus adding to the confusion.

Medical Devices/IDEs

The regulations require that all devices have an FDA-approved IDE for use in clinical research. A system, unique to devices, to comply with this regulation requires the determination by the reviewing IRB of whether the study presents a significant or non-significant risk to the subject population. A non-significant risk device study is considered to have an approved IDE application (i.e., no application need be filed with the FDA). With this non-significant risk determination, the study can be conducted without FDA oversight, as long as the device is properly labeled, has IRB approval, investigators obtain and document informed consent, proper study monitoring is conducted, and compliance is assured for all other IDE regulations. An FDA-approved IDE application is required prior to human subject exposure for all significant-risk device studies. Besides the IDE regulations, significant risk studies must comply with the IRB, informed consent, monitoring, and compliance regulations.

Although there is no Form FDA 1572 for device studies, documentation of similar commitments by the investigators is required in either the IDE application or in the sponsor's contracts with investigators. All investigators participating in studies with a significant risk device are to be listed in the IDE application.

Sponsor Responsibilities in FDA-Regulated Research

The study sponsor can be an individual, company, institution or other organization that takes responsibility for the initiation, management and financing of a research project or study. Investigators who also take on the role of sponsors must comply with the responsibilities of both roles.

The Responsibilities of the research sponsor can be divided into four main areas:

The Responsibilities of the research sponsor can be divided into four main areas:

1. Qualifying and Informing Investigators.

2. Monitoring of Study Conduct.

3. Completing Regulatory Filings.

4. Control of Product (Drug, Biologic or Device) Shipment and Disposition.

---

1. Qualifying and Informing Investigators

The sponsor is responsible for selecting and qualifying investigators. This involves reviewing the investigator's training and experience, and obtaining the investigator's commitment to:

- Conduct the study as agreed, including IRB stipulations.

- Supervise all testing.

- Obtain informed consent.

Once investigators are selected, the study sponsor is responsible for providing investigators with the necessary information to conduct the study, including reports of all prior investigations and the current investigational plan (protocol). Any additional significant information learned during the course of the study, including reports of adverse events from other sites, are to be provided to all investigators in timely manner. Information not critical to the conduct of a study may be provided at the time the investigator brochure is updated.

2. Monitoring of Study Conduct

Monitoring of studies is viewed as a critical step in securing compliance of all investigators and assuring that adequate subject informed consent is obtained. Any significant new safety information regarding study conduct must be provided to the reviewing IRB(s), the FDA and study investigators. It is the sponsor's responsibility to evaluate and terminate investigations if undue risks to study participants are observed.

For some NIH- and FDA-regulated studies, formal study monitors are appointed. The monitor reviews source documents to determine that reported data is accurate and complete. The monitor also audits the research to assure that the investigator is in compliance with:

- The approved protocol and amendments.

- Good Clinical Practices (GCPs).

- Applicable regulations.

3. Completing Regulatory Filings

It is the sponsor who must determine whether an application for an IDE or IND is necessary for a specific project. Once an exemption application is active, the sponsor is required to keep the FDA informed of any serious, related, unexpected adverse events, withdrawal of IRB approval for any reason, any recalls of test articles, progress reports (usually annually), any use of test articles without informed consent and a final study report.

For significant risk devices, the sponsor must also supply the FDA with a current list of investigators as well as any change in risk category. Sponsors are required to immediately conduct an evaluation of any unanticipated adverse device effect. If the sponsor determines that an unanticipated adverse device effect presents an unreasonable risk to study participants, then the sponsor must terminate all studies (or parts of the studies) that present that risk. This termination is to occur within five working days following sponsor determination, and no later than 15 working days after the sponsor first received notice of the effect. If the device is a significant-risk device, the sponsor may not resume a terminated study without reapproval from both the FDA and the IRB.

4. Control of Product (Drug, Biologic or Device) Shipment and Disposition

It is the sponsor's responsibility to control the distribution and disposition of all investigational test articles. Prior to the initial shipment, there must be documentation indicating that any necessary IDE or IND is filed and active and that the site's IRB has reviewed and approved the study. Test articles may only be shipped to qualified sites. Complete and accurate records are required for the shipment of test articles with an accounting of their final disposition.

> Prior to the initial shipment of test articles, there must be documentation indicating that the necessary IDE or IND is filed and active, and that the site's IRB has reviewed and approved the study.

The Study Process for Industry-Sponsored Studies

Clinical studies conducted on the behalf of industry sponsors are generally required to comply with Good Clinical Practices (GCPs), an international, ethical and scientific quality standard for designing, conducting, monitoring, recording, auditing, analyzing and reporting trials that involve participation of human subjects . The investigator responsibilities critical to the conduct of industry-sponsored studies include three additional processes.

1. Investigational Materials Handling and Accountability

For the purpose of this section, investigational materials are drugs or medical devices being tested in accordance with an approved protocol or investigational plan. The investigator is responsible for the accurate accountability and use of investigational materials provided to human subjects. By law, the investigator is required to maintain adequate records of the accountability and final disposition of the investigational drugs/devices.

Receipt, Handling and Storage of Investigational Materials

Upon receiving investigational materials, the investigator or appropriate staff member must adhere to the following:

- Verify the contents and integrity of each shipment against the packing slip and what materials were actually ordered.

- If no discrepancies are found, the investigator must acknowledge in writing to the sponsor the receipt of the materials. This is typically accomplished by signing the shipping document enclosed with the investigational materials. The investigator must notify the sponsor immediately if discrepancies are found.

- A copy of this receipt should be in the investigator's study file (or in pharmacy if the drug is received and dispensed there).

- All investigational materials must be stored in a secure (locked) limited access area.

    ⇨ Additionally, materials must be stored in accordance with the approved storage conditions (i.e., correct temperature, light and humidity).

Accountability Records

Drug or device accountability records (DARs) are used to provide evidence that, at the conclusion of the investigation, all materials are accounted for and that their final disposition is controlled (i.e., the materials are returned to the sponsor or destroyed). DARs (drug/device accountability records) are forms that are customized documents tailored to the individual protocol. The following minimum information should be captured on each form:

- Protocol Identification (protocol # and/or title).

- Principal investigator's name.

- Description of test article(s) received including batch or lot numbers.

- Date and time study drug/device dispensed/used.

- Amount dispensed (for drugs).

- Subject identification.

- Signature and/or initials of person dispensing the drug(s)/device(s).

- Amount returned by the subject, if any.

- Principal investigator's signature and date. [Note: The investigator should review, sign, and date the forms at the conclusion of the subject's participation in the trial.]

DARs may be created to track individual subjects enrolled in a trial or, in the case of small trials with single dose dispensing, may be customized to capture all participating subjects. The main objective of the regulations is to require the investigator to maintain adequate records of the disposition of the drug or device.

Drug / Device Returns (Final Disposition)

At the conclusion, discontinuance or termination of the study for both drugs and devices, the investigator is responsible for returning all unused medical devices and drugs to the trial sponsor. Return shipments should include a list of the contents, which must be reconciled with the amounts originally received and the amounts used by the subjects.

Alternatively, after drug/device accountability records are complete, the sponsor may authorize alternative disposition for these materials (destruction by the investigator). Any directive from the sponsor allowing destruction must be in writing. The investigator will be responsible for assuring that the destruction is carried out, and the investigator must maintain a written record of destruction.

2. Adverse Events

Drug and Biologic Requirements

All clinical investigators are required to report to the sponsor any adverse events that may be caused by the investigational product (the timeline is defined in the study protocol). The investigator is also required to report to the reviewing IRB any injury (harm caused by involvement in research), deaths and unexpected serious adverse experiences.

Device Requirements

The regulations require that investigators prepare and submit complete, accurate and timely reports of unanticipated adverse device effects to the sponsor and to the reviewing IRB as soon as possible, but no later than 15 calendar days after the investigator learns of the effect.

3. Documentation

Source Documentation

Investigators are required to prepare and maintain adequate and accurate records of all observations and other data pertinent to the study for each subject. Source documentation is where the information is first recorded, specifically original documents, data, and records (including medical records and case report forms).

> Source documentation is where the information is first recorded, including medical records and case report forms.

The investigator must maintain primary source documents supporting significant data for each subject in the case history records. These documents, which are considered 'source data,' should include documentation of the following:

- Demographic information.

- Evidence supporting the diagnosis/condition for which the subject is being studied.

- General information or medical history demonstrating that the subject meets the inclusion and exclusion criteria.

- Physical findings.

- Hospital records (if appropriate).

- Each study visit by date.

- Relevant findings/notes by the investigator.

- Occurrence (or lack of) adverse events.

- Changes in test article usage.

- Any relevant telephone conversations with the subject.

- Information regarding the subject's exposure to test or control article.

- Documentation that informed consent was obtained for each subject prior to participation in the study.

The investigator must also retain all printouts/test reports/procedures/forms for each subject. Examples include:

- Original, signed consent forms.

- Diagnostic test results, X-rays and laboratory test results.

- Subject diaries or evaluation checklists.

- Clinical and office charts.

- Consultations.

- Drug and device receipt, accountability and return records.

- Case report forms.

- Test instruments.

Investigators also need to maintain the following:

- Copies of all correspondence sent to or received by the study sponsor and the monitor.

- The protocol.

- Protocol amendments.

- Records of IRB communication and study approval.

- Materials used in recruiting subjects (e.g., flyers).

- Materials used in obtaining informed consent.

- Investigator brochure.

Case Report Forms

These forms are critical study documents. Study results are a summary of the data reported to the sponsor on case report forms. The case report form may or may not duplicate all information in the subject's case history. Case report forms may be printed or electronic documents. It is important that:

- The content of the case report forms capture data as required by the protocol.

- The investigator ensures the accuracy of the data recorded on the case report form.

> It is the responsibility of the investigator to ensure the accuracy of the data recorded on the case report form.

The ICH GCP guidelines specify that the protocol should identify any data to be recorded directly on the case report forms and classify what is considered to be source data. During monitoring visits, the monitor will validate data recorded on the case report forms against source data.

Record Retention

Investigators are required to retain all study records in a secure and safe facility with limited access until one of the following time periods:

- At least two years after notification from the sponsor that the drug/device has been approved for the indication that was investigated.

- Or, if not approved for such indication, at least two years after the investigation is completed or discontinued and the FDA has been notified by the sponsor.

> Investigators are advised to contact the study sponsor before any study records are destroyed to ensure compliance with the regulatory requirements.

The investigator should notify the sponsor of any change in the location, disposition or custody of the study files and are advised to contact the study sponsor before any study records are destroyed to ensure compliance with the regulatory requirements.

Sponsor-Investigator-Institution Interaction Issues

The interactions between the sponsor, investigator and institution (including the IRB) may be complex. Generally, the investigator provides the route of communication between the sponsor and institution, although direct contact may expedite resolution of certain issues.

An IRB is required to notify the investigator in writing of its decision to approve, disapprove or request modification to a research project. The investigator must provide the sponsor with a copy of this correspondence, since they are also responsible for ensuring that studies are conducted in compliance with informed consent and IRB regulations. Most sponsors will not ship the investigational product before they have all institutional approvals and other required paperwork.

Responsibilities of the Investigator-Sponsor

When there is no company or other organization acting as sponsor, individuals may become a sponsor of a clinical research study by assuming the roles and responsibilities of the study sponsor. For clinical investigators, this means that one individual is assuming all the responsibilities of the study sponsor in addition to that of investigator. The additional tasks of the sponsor include all of the regulatory reporting (FDA) requirements (see below), responsibility for drug manufacture and control issues (including proper labeling of the investigational product), the assessment of safety, ensuring IRB approval prior to shipping clinical supplies to sites, and informing and monitoring all investigators.

The scope of the regulatory filings vary with the intent of the project. If the data being collected are only for publication, the application is generally short. These projects are usually small studies. The FDA reviews these "non-commercial INDs" mainly for safety concerns.

For commercial development projects, the initial application is generally longer and more detailed. Detailed manufacturing information is required at each step, but especially as the project moves towards the larger efficacy trials (phase III). All protocols must be submitted for FDA and IRB review prior to study initiation. The FDA reviews these applications for both subject safety and for the ability to satisfy the statutory requirement for efficacy.

Original Application

The investigator-sponsor is responsible for filing adequate information in the initial IND or IDE application to allow the FDA to make a decision on whether the study risks are acceptable. The investigator-sponsor is required to wait 30 days for FDA review prior to enrolling subjects in the study. If no notice is received within that 30-day period that indicates that the FDA has concerns with the application, the IND or IDE is considered to be approved. It is advisable, however, to call the FDA to confirm that they do not have any issues or concerns with the application. Note that if insufficient information is filed, the FDA may place a clinical hold on the application. Absolutely no subjects are to be enrolled in the study until the FDA has removed all holds on an application. If the FDA denies the application, then the project may not be initiated. It is possible to reapply to the FDA for the same project, if modified to be acceptable to the FDA.

Amendments to Documentation

Any new clinical study protocol must be submitted under the IND/IDE prior to study initiation. This is true for changes to any other information within an application that has an impact on subject safety. These can be filed at any time, but before any human subjects are exposed. Minor changes that do not impact human subject safety may be submitted in the annual report.

IND Safety Reports

Investigator-sponsors are required to notify the FDA and all participating investigators in writing of any adverse experience that is **serious, related (associated) and unexpected.** This information may be submitted in a narrative format or on the FDA Form 3500A (the MedWatch form also used to report post-marketing adverse event information). The investigator-sponsor must also determine if any safety reports had previously been filed that are similar to each new reportable event. The significance of the new report must be analyzed with regard to previous, similar reports. The report must be clearly marked "IND Safety Report" and must be filed with the FDA no more than 15 calendar days after the investigator-sponsor initially receives the information. These reports are sent directly to the division of the FDA responsible for reviewing the IND.

The investigator-sponsor is to notify the FDA by telephone of any **unexpected, fatal or life-threatening experience** associated with the use of a drug in clinical studies conducted under the IND, within seven calendar days after receiving the information. For this purpose only, the FDA defines life-threatening as the subject being at *immediate* risk of death from the reaction.

> Serious, related, unexpected adverse experiences must be promptly reported to FDA.

Note that sponsors of INDs for marketed drugs are NOT required to report adverse events associated with the use of the drug that occur outside of the studies conducted under their INDs (i.e., literature reports and events reported during patient care are not reportable to the IND). However, if such information affects the perceived risks to the subjects in the clinical trials, the information needs to be shared with the investigators and their respective IRBs.

Definitions: The FDA provides the following definitions for reporting adverse events:

- *Associated with the use of the drug:* There is a reasonable possibility that the experience may have been caused by the drug.

- *Disability:* A substantial disruption of a person's ability to conduct normal life functions.

- *Life threatening adverse drug experience:* Any adverse drug experience that places the subject, in the view of the investigator, at immediate risk of death from the reaction as it occurred, i.e., it does not include a reaction, had it occurred in a more severe form, which might have caused death.

- *Unexpected adverse drug experience:* Any adverse experience, the specificity or severity of which is not consistent with the current investigator brochure or package insert; or not consistent with the risk information described in the general investigational plan or elsewhere in the current application.

- *Serious adverse drug experience:* Any adverse drug experience occurring at any dose that results in any of the following outcomes:

  ⇨ Death.

  ⇨ A life-threatening adverse experience.

  ⇨ Hospitalization or prolongation of existing hospitalization.

  ⇨ A persistent or significant disability/incapacity.

  ⇨ Or a congenital anomaly or birth defect.

Important medical events that may not result in death, be life threatening or require hospitalization may be considered serious adverse drug experiences when, based upon medical judgment, they jeopardize the subject and may require medical or surgical intervention to prevent one of the outcomes listed in this definition. [Note: Data from animal studies are also reportable as IND Safety Reports if any serious adverse drug experience is observed that suggests a significant risk for human subjects, including any finding of mutagenicity, teratogenicity or carcinogenicity.]

Unanticipated Adverse Device Effect Reports: The reporting requirements for adverse device effects are different from those for drugs and biologics. The sponsor-investigator must immediately conduct an evaluation of any unanticipated adverse device effect. If this effect presents an unreasonable risk to subjects, the sponsor-investigator is required to terminate all investigations as soon as possible, but no later than five working days after the sponsor makes this determination. This also must occur within 15 working days of when the sponsor was notified for the adverse effect.

Both the FDA and the IRB must be informed of unanticipated adverse device effects. Any terminated study must NOT be resumed without approval of both the FDA and the reviewing IRB.

Annual Reports

An annual report is required for INDs and IDEs. It is due no later than 60 calendar days after the anniversary date of an application going into effect.

The format for the annual report is provided in regulatory guidance documents. Critical components of these reports include:

- Protocol summaries, for ongoing and completed studies, to document the total human exposure under the application.

- All changes made to protocols or manufacturing information. This is the mechanism to report minor changes that occurred during the year that were not subject to amendments.

- New pre-clinical (animal) and clinical information. Any impact on human subject safety should be addressed.

- Changes to the investigational plan for the coming year.

- Any information requested, but not received, from the FDA should also be documented.

Final Study Reports

The regulations require that a final report be written and submitted for all clinical studies. This report should be submitted within six months of study completion.

Withdrawal of Application

Upon completion of studies, when no additional work is envisioned, the investigator-sponsor should send a letter to the FDA requesting withdrawal of the IND/IDE.

Additional Issues to Consider for Investigator-Sponsors

IRB Approval at Study Sites: A copy of the IRB approval letter should be obtained from each study site prior to the shipment of any investigational materials. For device studies, the determination of significant versus non-significant risk should be documented. Verbal assurance of submission to an IRB should not be considered adequate.

Liability Concerns: For industry sponsored studies, the company, the institution and the investigator share responsibility for research study-related injury to study subjects. For investigator-sponsored studies, the liability for research-related injury lies completely with the investigator and associated institution.

Conflict of Interest: There may be a conflict of interest for investigator-sponsors, especially where financial or career enhancement benefits exist with a project. Documentation of all financial compensation is required by the FDA prior to approving products for market.

Contracts: Investigator-sponsors must have all contracts related to the conduct of research reviewed and approved by the appropriate institutional office.

Clinical Supplies: Obtaining appropriate clinical supplies for research is the responsibility of the study sponsor. Manufacturing issues are of concern to the FDA when reviewing non-commercial or commercial applications. When pharmaceutical-grade material is not available, documentation of product identity, purity and lack of contamination is generally required. This usually involves testing of each batch of clinical supplies by a qualified laboratory.

BEHAVIORAL RESEARCH ISSUES

Objectives

At the conclusion of this chapter, readers will be able to:

- Describe the potential risks associated with behavioral research.
- Discuss privacy and confidentiality issues.
- Explain the issues around deception.

Introduction

When people think of research, especially research risk, often they think only of medical research. This is due to the fact that much of the focus on research and research ethics has been on the dangers posed by biomedical research and the harms caused by transgressions of researchers in that field. However, research with drugs, devices and other medical procedures is only a part of the total research endeavor. Many studies are also conducted in human behavior, social science, education, anthropology, epidemiology and similar areas. For brevity, these will be subsumed here under the broad label 'behavioral research.' The following issues are also important for bio-medical researchers as many of the concerns may be present to some extent in those studies as well.

Federal Regulations

The federal regulations governing research have included behavioral research from the start. In recognition that these studies often present only slight risks, the regulations allow some activities to be exempt from regulation and others to be given a brief review. This does not imply a lesser standard for these studies, but rather an increased reliance on the investigator to conduct the study within appropriate ethical and scientific bounds. Investigators who believe their research is exempt should check with the IRB to verify that an exemption applies. Exemptions may be granted for some studies in the following categories:

- Activities that use research methods, but are not "research" according to federal definitions (e.g., quality assurance studies and in-house program evaluations).

- Research that does not involve 'human subjects.'

- Educational research conducted in normal educational settings.

- Survey/interview/observational research with adults.

- Secondary use of pre-existing data.

- Evaluation of public benefit or service programs.

- Taste and food quality studies.

Psychological/Social Risks

Because there often is no physical intervention, these studies do not generally pose a risk to physical well-being, but they do carry risks of their own. The main points of concern are with other types of potential harms such as psychological, social, economic and legal. These risks may be as harmful as any risk faced by a subject in a medical study. Humans are by nature introspective, and reflecting upon the actions we have or have not taken may cause us emotional pain. While taking a course of action based upon wrong or incomplete information may make it easier to rationalize that action, discovering that we are capable of violating societal and/or our own standards can be psychologically damaging, as in the Milgram study.

Psychological hazards run from temporary anxiety and distress to relapse and precipitation of behavioral disorders. Social harms include both direct personal impacts such as embarrassment, ostracism, stigmatization and loss of status as well as similar effects upon the subject's family and community. Risks in the economic area include job loss and decreased employability. Legal risks include arrest, prosecution and civil or criminal liability.

Exposure to risks of biomedical research are typically faced only by the individual. In behavioral research, however, the range of non-physical risks above may have an impact on others including families, social groups, communities, ethnic populations and even entire societies. Prevailing community attitudes are an important consideration in the acceptability of behavioral research. Likewise, the investigator must be responsible in the use of research findings.

Therefore, in assessing the risks presented by a study, investigators, IRBs and subjects must consider a wide range of potential harms. Investigators should anticipate potential problem areas and design the study to provide an adequate level of protection. The traditional risk/benefit balance is also somewhat changed as the benefits rarely accrue to the individual subject, but rather to science and/or society.

Deception

Deception in research is intentionally misleading subjects or withholding full information about the nature of the experiment. Deception may take the form of covert observation or failing to fully inform the subject when obtaining consent. Misleading or omitted information might include the purpose of the research, the role of the investigator or what procedures are actually experimental. Deception interferes with the subject's ability to give informed consent. As such, it can be thought of as a wrong in itself, as a limiting influence on the protection afforded by informed consent and a violation of the norms of trust and truthfulness. Ethical concerns are increased whenever the protection of informed consent is compromised in any way because the research subjects are deprived of the opportunity to protect their own interests.

For certain types of behavioral inquiry, deception is arguably necessary because humans act differently depending on circumstances, and the subject's full knowledge would thus bias the results. Federal regulations (Common Rule) permit, but establish limitations, on the use of deception. Use of deception must be scientifically and ethically justified and approved by an IRB. In cases where the study can only be conducted with subjects who are less than fully informed, the missing information should not increase the risks of the study. After the experiment is conducted, subjects should be fully debriefed. This can be a formal process that includes assessment of the subject's reaction to the deception, or an informal discussion. In any event, subjects must have the opportunity to ask questions about the new information and be given the opportunity to withdraw from the study and have their data removed as well. It is not permissible to use deception to obtain enrollments.

Vulnerable Subjects

People are autonomous when they can deliberate personal goals and act accordingly. The capacity for self-determination increases with maturity. Individuals may lose this capacity because of physical illness, mental disability or while under circumstances that severely restrict liberty. The regulations define as 'vulnerable populations' those groups that may contain some individuals who have limited autonomy, i.e., they can not give informed consent. Such groups include children, some mentally disabled, individuals with dementia and other cognitive disorders and prisoners. The regulations require that IRBs treat pregnant women as a vulnerable population because of the need to avoid unnecessary risk to the fetus and because of the additional health concerns during pregnancy. Additional protections when conducting research with these populations may include the use of witnesses, requiring consultants/advocates, formally renewing consent at specified stages and limiting the scope of research projects.

Privacy and Confidentiality

An area that generally creates more concern for behavioral research than for biomedical studies is confidentiality and privacy. In fact, these concerns are often the central considerations for behavioral research. A major tenet in the protection of human subjects is that persons can be wronged even if they are not harmed. This philosophy focuses upon rights, both individual and societal. We have a right to expect that our private actions will remain private and that information others have about us will be kept confidential and only used for their original purposes (e.g., medical care or college admission). A related concern that will not be addressed here is the public debate about the appropriateness of scientific inquiry into areas considered by society to be private (e.g., sex and drug use). These are of concern because the results of social research can impact the core values and the support programs of society at large.

> A major tenet in the protection of human subjects is that persons can be wronged even if they are not harmed.

Privacy is itself a form of personal protection. So, a violation of an individual's privacy not only is a harm itself but also may cause the loss of this protective barrier. Risks include public exposure, perceived loss of control of person and a sense of insecurity. Breaches of privacy also erode trust on all levels.

These are concerns for behavioral studies that observe otherwise private behaviors or obtain private confidential information. Investigators must design studies to maximize data confidentiality to avoid unintentional release or other disclosures. Investigators should avoid violations of privacy, for example, by removing identifiers or using anonymous data. Certificates of confidentiality may be obtained from DHHS to protect study data from involuntary disclosure through subpoena.

Study Methods

The diversity in research topics and the research methods appropriate to those studies are unique features in the field of behavioral research. Study methods used include surveys, interviews, questionnaires, record reviews, observation (participatory, overt or covert) and various psychological and social interventions in laboratory and field settings, to mention a few. Each method itself presents ethical and scientific considerations.

> Every research method presents unique ethical and
> scientific considerations.

Laboratory and field experimentation may have no concerns in the areas of privacy and confidentiality but may involve consent issues and the full range of research risks. Survey and interview research may be just the reverse, that is, no concerns regarding consent but possible confidentiality concerns. Record reviews may raise both consent and privacy issues. Thus, investigators must design studies with an eye to minimizing the negative effects of the study's methods themselves.

Quality of Life Issues

Although not a "behavioral" issue in the strict sense, investigators should be aware of the possible effects of studies on the daily life of subjects. The demands of participation in studies can seriously disrupt the flow of normal activities. Side effects and even successful outcome of bio-medical studies may lead to a decrease in the quality of life (for example, by prolonged pain and suffering). As indicated above, even surveys can potentially cause psychological stress that may lead to long-term disabilities and a decline in aspects of lifestyle. Investigators need to design studies that take into consideration quality of life issues and they need to ensure potential subjects understand potential impacts on their personal lifestyle.

Points to Consider

When designing and conducting research, investigators should consider the following items:

- Minimize the potential for stress, discomfort and other harms.

- Use deception only when absolutely necessary and then follow with complete debriefing.

- Search for alternatives to deception.

- Respect subjects' privacy and minimize intrusion.

- Design mechanisms to protect confidentiality of data.

- Guard against factors leading to undue influence.

- Provide adequate safeguards when studying vulnerable populations.

CHAPTER 7

PUBLICATION OF STUDY RESULTS

Objectives

At the conclusion of this chapter, readers will be able to:

- Explain why investigators, administrators and organization sponsors may have different expectations for publishing and presenting data.

- Discuss the implications of publishing study results for the investigator, the sponsor, other researchers and the public.

- Identify and minimize potential areas of conflict before starting the study.

Introduction

Surveys show that professionals at the graduate and post-graduate levels receive most of their new knowledge by reading, especially the current peer-reviewed periodicals. Thus, it is important that research be published in a timely manner, in an appropriate venue, and that data be presented accurately and clearly. Most of the time, this is the case. However, scientific publication is not immune to fraud and misconduct.

In his book, *Stealing into Print (1992)*, Marcel Lafollette defines fraud in scientific communication as "...when an author, editor or referee makes a false representation to obtain some unfair advantage or to injure deliberately the rights or interests of another person or group." This may include any of the following:

- Presenting data that do not exist or have been "made up."

- Misrepresenting or deliberately altering evidence.

- Plagiarism.

- Misrepresentation of authorship.

- Unreasonably delaying review or publication for personal gain.

The underlying reasons for such actions may be personal (e.g., fame, career advancement, institutional pressure to publish) or financial (i.e., monetary gain, investment options, competitive advantage in the market). Another reason is the conflict of interest that may occur between the investigator and the source of funding for the research. This type of conflict directly challenges the accountability and independence of the investigator and can create considerable tension between the investigator, the sponsor and the institution where the research is being done. This chapter reviews some of the key issues for scientific publication related to conflicts of interest between sponsor and investigator.

> Professionals receive most of their new knowledge by reading, especially the current peer-reviewed periodicals. Research results should be published in a timely manner and in an appropriate venue.

Examples of fraud in scientific publication can be found in all fields – from archaeology to psychology to engineering and medicine. However, in terms of press coverage, it is misconduct within the biomedical arena that receives the most attention. This probably relates to two factors: 1) there is greater public awareness and interest in matters of health; and 2) more sponsored funding is available from government agencies and from the pharmaceutical and biotechnology industries. Thus, the cases presented in this chapter focus on biomedical research, specifically research sponsored by industry. However, the issues and principles illustrated are not unique to medicine or biology but are applicable to any type of academic research funded by an outside source.

There are no federal regulations governing the dissemination of research results. However, at least one government agency, the Food and Drug Administration (FDA), has published guidelines addressing the dissemination of industry-sponsored research. The FDA does not object to a company providing financial support to an investigator to present data or to publish a manuscript but notes that there may be questions regarding the circumstances that may occur in such an arrangement. For example, there may be questions regarding independence: Will the investigator-author actually write the article or will the sponsor provide assistance in the way of a medical writer? If the latter, how much input will the investigator actually have? There also may be issues around the timing of the publication: Could the sponsor try to delay (or, in extreme cases, even stop) publication of the data if they are not "acceptable" to them? The answers to these questions are not always as straightforward as they might seem. Two cases can serve as illustrations.

> FDA concerns about publishing industry-sponsored studies most frequently focus on independence and how the sponsor may affect independence.

Case One: B. Dong v. Boots Pharmaceuticals

In the April 16, 1997 issue of the *Journal of the American Medical Association* (JAMA), Dong et al (University of California at San Francisco) reported a study of the bioequivalence of generic and branded levothyroxine products in the treatment of hypothyroidism. Two generic products (Geneva Generics; Rugby) were compared with two brand-name medications (Synthroid, Boots Pharmaceuticals [now Knoll Pharmaceuticals]; Levoxine [now Levoxyl] Daniels Pharmaceuticals, Inc. [now Jones Medical Industries]) using current FDA criteria for bioequivalence. The study was funded, in part, by Flint Laboratories (which was taken over by Boots Pharmaceuticals during the course of the study), the manufacturers of Synthroid. As is usual for this type of sponsorship, Dr. Dong signed a contract with Flint Laboratories. Company representatives made regular site visits, and copies of the data were sent to the manufacturer.

Preliminary analysis of the data indicated that all four medications were bioequivalent according to the FDA standards for oral preparations, thereby implying that the products were clinically interchangeable. In reviewing the results, the investigators calculated that if the generics or the other brand-name preparation were substituted for Synthroid, $356 million might be saved annually. These results were obtained in 1990, yet the published report did not appear until 1997. What happened between 1990 and 1997 that delayed publication?

Obviously, the sponsor and the investigators had conflicting views about publication of the results. The investigators believed that the results had important clinical implications and should be shared with the medical and academic community. The sponsor, on the other hand, was concerned that the results would increase market share for the generic products at the expense of the brand-name product. In this case, the sponsor attempted to prevent publication. The company complained to administrators at UCSF that procedures were not carried out as detailed in the protocol, and they suggested that the results were flawed due to problems with patient selection, compliance, assay reliability and statistical analysis. UCSF responded to the complaints with an internal investigation that revealed no major problems with the study. They concluded that the study was rigorously conducted in a way that complied fully with the contract; and they supported publication. Responding to the company after almost four years of review, UCSF noted that all data had been open to the sponsor and that the sponsor had monitored the study closely. Thus, the University concluded that there was no reason to suppress the manuscript, and that to do so would be "an unprecedented intrusion upon academic freedom."

> Suppressing publication of study results can be viewed as an intrusion upon academic freedom. However, industry sponsors may have other concerns (e.g. patent infringement, commercial interests, liability issues).

Dr. Dong submitted the manuscript to JAMA in April 1994, along with a letter disclosing the funding of the study and the criticism from the sponsor. Publication was originally intended for early 1995, when Dr. Dong abruptly withdrew the manuscript from the journal due to "impending legal action by Boots Pharmaceutical, Inc. against UCSF and the investigators." The basis for the legal action was the following contract clause: "All information contained in this protocol is confidential and is to be used by the investigator only for the conduct of this study. Data obtained by the investigator while carrying out this study is also considered confidential and *is not to be published or otherwise released without written consent from Flint Laboratories, Inc.*" UCSF did not have this permission, and a University attorney indicated that the authors could not be defended if a suit ensued.

Interestingly, the University of California, like most universities in the United States, prohibits restrictions on publishing rights. In fact, the UCSF contract of employment (signed by Dr. Dong) stated that "...the University will undertake research or studies *only if the scientific results can be published or otherwise promptly disseminated,...*" So, how did this happen? The fact is that protocol contracts with pharmaceutical sponsors often contain restrictive clauses, yet rarely have they prevented publication. Dr. Dong and her colleagues believed that these contracts, regardless of content, could not prevent publication.

> Protocol contracts with industry sponsors may contain restrictive clauses. Pay attention to confidentiality clauses that prohibit publication without permission from the sponsor.

The issue came to the attention of the public on April 25, 1996, when an article appeared in the *Wall Street Journal*. In the article, Carter Eckert (president, Boots Pharmaceuticals) was quoted, "I stopped a flawed study that would have put millions of patients at risk." Additionally, in 1994, Boots, now Knoll, had received a letter from the FDA stating that a manuscript published by company researchers in 1992 was misleading, and that dissemination of the article by the company should cease. The conclusions of this paper opposed those of Dr. Dong , namely that in normal volunteers studied over 48 hours, the bioavailability of Synthroid was superior to Levoxine. The FDA commented that the study design was not appropriate for comparing bioequivalence, noting specifically that "…a more complex design involving chronic administration in a well-controlled, hypothyroid population with the measurement of several endpoints would be required" (precisely the protocol used by Dong and her colleagues). In their response to the FDA, Knoll referred to the work by Dr. Dong, but dismissed it as "worthless." However, the FDA took exception, writing that the Dong study was appropriate to test bioequivalence and cited Knoll for not previously disclosing the Dong results.

Under pressure from the FDA and scrutiny from the public, Knoll ultimately agreed to publication of the manuscript. JAMA published the paper along with letters from Knoll apologizing for the delay and objecting to the findings. Rebuttals from the investigator/authors were also published. The cost calculations were included in the discussion. The accompanying comments of the journal editors are of particular interest:

> *We do not claim that we are publishing a perfect study, just one of the best, made as good as expert review can make it. Experience has taught us that there are very few studies in which some reviewers cannot find flaws… it is our belief that this is a good study carried out by highly competent workers following a sensible design that tried to answer an important question. It is hard to believe that the sponsors would have made such extraordinary efforts to delay and block publication of the study for such a very long time and for such an extraordinary number of specious reasons if the results had shown Synthroid to be better.*

Case Two: D. Kern v. Microfibres, Inc.

The second case involves an agreement for services between industry and a physician/investigator/consultant. The services in this case, were provided by Dr. David Kern, an associate professor at Brown University School of Medicine and Chief of General Internal Medicine and Director of Occupational and Environmental Health Service (OEHS) at the Memorial Hospital of Rhode Island. In his latter role, Dr. Kern provided consultancy services, as needed, to local industry and agencies regarding occupational and environmental health hazards.

Over a two year period, in the early 1990s, the OEHS identified two cases of interstitial lung disease (ILD). Reviewing the cases, Dr. Kern noted that both patients had been employees of a local textile plant, Microfibres, Inc (Pawtucket, R.I.). As is required by health regulations in the United States, Dr. Kern notified the company and then reviewed company health records. He found that there had been a similar "outbreak" of ILD cases at the company's Canadian facility in 1990, and notified the National Institute for Occupational Safety and Health (NIOSH). Additionally, Dr. Kern approached company officials, offering his services as a consultant to study the ILD outbreaks. The company agreed, and Dr. Kern signed a confidentiality agreement. The ensuing review identified another six "work-related" cases of ILD in 150 employees.

In the summer of 1996, Dr. Kern prepared an abstract of his findings for submission to the 1997 annual meeting of the American Thoracic Society (ATS). Prior to submission, Dr. Kern shared copies of the abstract with both company and hospital officials. Microfibres responded that the information was confidential and should not be submitted. They cited the consultancy agreement that Dr. Kern had signed, which included a clause about the protection of "trade secrets." The company threatened a lawsuit if the abstract was submitted and notified administrators at both the hospital and the medical school. Dr. Kern's position was that the data was of public health interest, and he assured the officials that publication and/or presentation of the data would not include any proprietary information. He appealed to the Dean of Medicine at Brown University at the end of October 1996 to help him in this academic freedom issue; however, the school was slow to act. Meanwhile, Dr. Kern submitted the abstract, and presented the data as a poster at the May 1997 annual meeting of the American Thoracic Society (ATS).

> Sponsors and investigators may have conflicting perspectives on what constitutes a "trade secret." Open communication BEFORE signing agreements is important.

In December 1996, the Memorial Hospital of Rhode Island closed the OEHS. In May 1997, following the ATS meeting, Dr. Kern was notified that his employment at the hospital would not be renewed when his contract expired. At this point, Dr. Kern went to the academic community at Brown University, submitting the documents for their review. Writing to his colleagues, he noted that:

> As an Associate Professor of Medicine at Brown... I have waited patiently these last six months for the University administration to intervene on the side of academic freedom, professional ethics and public health. I have waited in vain.

The faculty appealed to the President of Brown University. Independently, the issue was also brought forward by Brown's Faculty Executive Committee (FEC). In the end, the President obtained an agreement from the hospital allowing Dr. Kern to continue his program, grants and contracts until at least 2000.

Interestingly, administration at Brown continues to maintain that Dr. Kern's academic freedom had not been violated as it was he who decided to publish. The lesson learned, according to the FEC, is that it is the faculty and not the administration who are the "watchdogs" of academic freedom.

Withholding Data

Withholding or delaying the publication or presentation of research results is defined as not publishing or presenting the data for at least six months after completion of the study. It is not only the sponsor who may attempt to delay the dissemination of research data. In fact, when data are withheld, it is most often the investigator who has chosen to do so. This was one of the conclusions of a survey of 3,394 life science faculty in 50 universities in the United States. The universities were identified according to the amount of NIH funding received in 1993: the top 50 were included in the survey.

Approximately 20% of 2,100 researchers who responded to the survey indicated that they had delayed the publication of study results in the past. The majority of the researchers had delayed publication in order to protect the commercial value of the data: 46% cited the time for patent application as a reason; another 33% cited other proprietary and/or financial value of the data; and 26% had delayed publication due to the time needed for licensing. Other common reasons given were to protect their own scientific lead, reported by 46% of the researchers (and often attributed to increased competition for funding), and to delay the publication of "undesirable" results, reported by 28% of the researchers surveyed.

Only 4% of the researchers reported that dissemination of study results had been delayed due to any formal agreement with an industry sponsor. Other reasons included avoiding potential liability issues.

The reasons given by investigators for withholding or delaying the dissemination of data are very similar to the reasons given by companies. However, in addition, a company may delay publication in order to avoid artificial inflation of stock or to wait for FDA approval of a new product or new indication so that claims of efficacy and safety can be made appropriately.

Lessons to be Learned From These Cases

These two cases provide classic illustrations of the tension that can develop between industry sponsors and investigators due to different interpretations of what is in contracts and consultancy agreements, and also due to different expectations of what will happen to the data once the study is concluded.

Tension between investigators and industry may occur due to:

- Different interpretations of contractual text.

- Different expectations of what will happen to the data.

The Research Contract and Consultancy Agreement

Both cases could have been avoided if the investigator/consultant had carefully read the contract and asked for clarification of key points. Some take-away messages that may be important for investigators/consultants are:

- Read the contract! Know exactly what you are signing.

- Obtain the proper institutional reviews/approvals of the grant/contract.

- Ask the sponsor questions. Do not assume that your interpretation of "trade secret," "proprietary information" or "confidential information" matches that of the sponsor. Ask the sponsor to define these terms explicitly. If your interpretation and their interpretation differ, then there should be an open discussion. Most industry sponsors are very open to these types of discussions and negotiations. If the sponsor is not willing to negotiate, get assistance with (or avoid) the agreement.

- Know your rights. This means knowing your institution's policies. What is the perspective of the institution regarding industry sponsors? If a lawsuit ensues between you and the sponsor, will the institution defend you? Are there any situations in which the institution may not legally be able to defend you?

- Before signing any agreement, review your employment contract. Specifically, look for any terms that negate points included in the company agreement.

- Recognize the different concerns of all parties involved – yourself, your colleagues who may be working with you on the project, your institution and the sponsor.

- Remember that if you sign a contract without carefully reviewing it, you may be signing away certain rights, including your right to legal defense by your institution.

> Carnegie Mellon University reported that 35% of signed agreements between universities and industry sponsors allowed the sponsor to delete information from publication, 53% allowed publication to be delayed, and 30% allowed both.

The Data

> **Three steps to prevent contract conflicts:**
>
> - Read the contract. Know exactly what you are signing.
> - Ask questions. Clarify all issues and terminology.
> - Know your rights.

It is important to clarify what data are and who controls the data. Different academic institutions have different definitions of what data are, for legal reasons.

> All contracts must be approved by the institution before you sign them.

Research data may be created through programs funded by external sponsors (e.g., government agencies, industry, private foundations). However, regardless of the funding, it is the institution that usually holds title to, or "owns," the data produced. The "creator(s)" of the data (i.e., the investigators) and the sponsors of the research retain rights to access and use of the data. To avoid situations such as those faced by Dr. Dong and her colleagues, know how your institution defines data and what the institution's perspective is regarding publication and presentation.

- Read the contract carefully, particularly terms that affect the publication and dissemination of the study results. Do not sign until any issues that you have are addressed by the institution and the sponsor.

- Do not assume that sponsors will encourage (or even permit) publication of unfavorable results.

- Do not allow sponsors veto power for publication or presentation of data.

- Know the position of your institution regarding restrictive clauses in relation to the publication and dissemination of data.

- Ask questions about the intentions of the sponsor with regard to publication and dissemination of the results. Consider asking the following questions:

    ⇨ Will this data be published? Will it be published if it is equivocal or negative?

    ⇨ Who will write the publication?

    ⇨ What other studies has the sponsor recently completed? Were the data published? If so, where and how long after the study was conducted?

    ⇨ When will the data be published?

    ⇨ Will the publication be limited by any concerns regarding potential claims and fair balance?

    ⇨ Are there financial or commercial interests at stake in the results? Will publication of the data have potential impact on these interests?

- Be honest about your expectations regarding the presentation and publication of study results.

Summary

Sponsors come to researchers at academic institutions in order to establish mutually beneficial and cooperative relationships. They are attracted by the institution's reputation, credibility and prestige. Most sponsors know that academic investigators need to report study results, and that there is a high premium placed on publication.

It is in the long-term interest of sponsors of research at academic institutions to not include restrictive clauses in their contracts that could affect the dissemination of study results. Sponsors should recognize that results may or may not support the initial hypothesis, and that researchers need to present and publish studies in a timely manner. The investigator/consultant needs to recognize that the sponsor may have legitimate concerns regarding the timing of releasing data to publication: e.g., they may be awaiting FDA approval; there may be potential liability issues; publication might artificially inflate the stock price. Open discussion of the concerns of both parties *before* an agreement is signed will prevent situations that compromise the credibility of either.

Finally, conflict of interest in the scientific publication of sponsored research is not limited to industry funding. There are published reports of similar cases involving professional societies and government agencies. A well-known example is the restrictions placed by the federal government on publishing data that might impact national security. The conflict arises when the definition of national security and perceptions of "impacting data" are not clearly communicated. Again, open and clear discussion between the sponsor, the researcher and the institution prior to signing an agreement will reduce the likelihood of potential disputes.

REFERENCES, RESOURCES AND SUGGESTED READINGS

CHAPTER ONE: Historical Perspectives on Human Subject Research

Annas G, Grodin M, eds. *The Nazi Doctors and the Nuremberg Code: Human Rights in Human Experimentation.* New York, NY: Oxford University Press, 1992.

Beecher HK. *Ethics and Clinical Research.* N Engl J Med 1996;274: 1354-60.

Caplan A, ed. *When Medicine Went Mad: Bioethics and the Holocaust.* Totowa, NJ: Humanna Press, 1992.

Faden R, ed. *Human Radiation Experiments: Final Report of the President's Advisory Committee.* New York, NY: Oxford University Press, 1996.

Faden R, Beauchamp T. *A History and Theory of Informed Consent.* New York, NY: Oxford University Press, 1986.

Jones J. *Bad Blood: The Tuskegee Syphilis Experiment.* New York, NY: Free Press, 1993.

Milgram S. *Obedience to Authority.* New York, NY: Harper & Row Publishers, Inc., 1974.

Third Report of the Attorney General's Research Working Group. Office of the Maryland Attorney General, Annapolis MD: Office of the Attorney General, August 1997.

CHAPTER TWO: Ethics and Federal Regulations

Belmont Report: Ethical Principles and Guidelines for the Protection of Human Subjects of Research. Federal Register Document 79-12065 (see: www.nih.gov/grants/oprr/humansubjects/guidance/belmont.htm).

Beauchamp TL, Childress JF. *Principles of Biomedical Ethics (4th ed.).* New York, NY: Oxford University Press, 1994.

Food, Drug, & Cosmetic Act (see: www.fda.gov).

Levine RJ. *Ethics and Regulation of Clinical Research (2nd ed.).* New Haven, CT: Yale University Press, 1986.

Office of Research Integrity (see: http://ori.dhhs.gov).

Office for Protection from Research Risks (OPRR) (see: http://www.nih.gov/grants/oprr/oprr.htm).

OPRR IRB Guidebook: Protecting Human Research Subjects. Washington, DC,: Government Printing Office, 1993.

CHAPTER THREE: Roles and Responsibilities of Institutions in Human Subject Research

21 Code of Federal Regulations (CFR) 312, 314, 812 and 814.

Food and Drug Administration (see: www.FDA.gov).

Food, Drug and Cosmetic Act (see: www.fda.gov).

National Institutes of Health (see: www.NIH.gov).

Research Subjects Review Board (see: www.urmc.rochester.edu/urmc/rsrb).

CHAPTER FOUR: The Roles and Responsibilities of the Investigator and the Study Process

FDA Clinical Investigator and IRB Information Sheets (see: www.FDA.gov).

Harwood F. *A Professional's Guide to ACP's Certification Program For Clinical Research Associates and Clinical Research Coordinators.* Washington, DC: Associates of Clinical Research Professionals (ACRP).

ICH Harmonized Tripartite Guideline: Guideline For Good Clinical Practice. (see: http://www.ifpma.org/pdfifpma/e6.pdf.).

Mackintosh DR, Zepp VJ. *GCP Responsibilities of Investigators-Beyond the 1572.* Appl Clin Trials. 1996; 5:32-40.

Sayre JE. GCP *Quality Audit Manual (1ˢᵗ ed.).* Buffalo Grove, IL: Interpharm Press; 1990.

Stephen L, Papke *A. Certified Clinical Research Coordinators.* Appl Clin Trials 1995; 4:58-63.

CHAPTER FIVE: FDA-Regulated Research Issues

21 CFR 312, 314, 812 and 814.

21 CFR 803 (Investigational Devices), 600 (Postmarketing), 310 (Investigational Drugs and Biologics).

Food and Drug Administration (see: www.FDA.gov).

Mackintosh DR, Zepp VJ. *GCP Responsibilities of Investigators-Beyond the 1572.* Appl Clin Trials. 1996; 5:32-40.

MEDWATCH: The FDA Medical Products Reporting Program

O'Donnell P. *Closer to Harmonized GCP.* Appl Clin Trials 1995; 4:48-53.

CHAPTER SIX: Behavioral Research Issues

Beauchamp, TL, Faden RR, Wallace RJ, et al. *Ethical Issues in Social Science Research.* Baltimore, MD: Johns Hopkins University Press.

OPRR IRB Guidebook: Protecting Human Research Subjects. Washington, DC: Government Printing Office, 1993.

CHAPTER SEVEN: Publications of Study Results

Berg JA, Mayor GH. *A study in normal human volunteers to compare the rate and extent of levothyroxine absorption from Synthroid and Levoxine.* J Clin Pharmacol 1992; 32:1135-40.

Blumenthal D, Campbell EG, Anderson MS, et al. *Withholding research results by academic life scientists: evidence from a national survey of faculty.* JAMA 1997; 277:1224-1228.

Cohen W, Florida R, Goe WR. *University-industry research centers in the United States.* Pittsburgh, PA: Carnegie Mellon University Press, 1994.

Committee on Science, Engineering, and Public Policy. *On Being A Scientist: Responsible Conduct in Research, (2nd edition)*. Washington, DC: National Academy of Sciences, National Academy of Engineering, Institute of Medicine, National Academy Press, 1995.

Dong BJ, Harck WW, Gambertoglio JG, et al. *Bioequivalence of generic and brand-name levothyroxine products in the treatment of hypothyroidism*. JAMA 1997; 277:1205-1213.

King R. *Bitter pill: how a drug company paid for university study, then undermined it*. Wall Street Journal. April 25, 1996:1.

LaFollette MC. *Stealing into Print*. Los Angeles, CA: University of California Press, 1992.

Rennie D. *Thyroid storm*. JAMA 1997; 277:1238-1243.

THE BELMONT REPORT

ETHICAL PRINCIPLES & GUIDELINES FOR RESEARCH INVOLVING HUMAN SUBJECTS

Scientific research has produced substantial social benefits. It has also posed some troubling ethical questions. Public attention was drawn to these questions by reported abuses of human subjects in biomedical experiments, especially during the Second World War. During the Nuremberg War Crime Trials, the Nuremberg code was drafted as a set of standards for judging physicians and scientists who had conducted biomedical experiments on concentration camp prisoners. This code became the prototype of many later codes[1] intended to assure that research involving human subjects would be carried out in an ethical manner.

The codes consist of rules, some general, others specific, that guide the investigators or the reviewers of research in their work. Such rules often are inadequate to cover complex situations; at times they come into conflict, and they are frequently difficult to interpret or apply. Broader ethical principles will provide a basis on which specific rules may be formulated, criticized and interpreted.

Three principles, or general prescriptive judgments, that are relevant to research involving human subjects are identified in this statement. Other principles may also be relevant. These three are comprehensive, however, and are stated at a level of generalization that should assist scientists, subjects, reviewers and interested citizens to understand the ethical issues inherent in research involving human subjects. These principles cannot always be applied so as to resolve beyond dispute particular ethical problems. The objective is to provide an analytical framework that will guide the resolution of ethical problems arising from research involving human subjects.

This statement consists of a distinction between research and practice, a discussion of the three basic ethical principles, and remarks about the application of these principles.

Part A: Boundaries Between Practice & Research

A. Boundaries Between Practice and Research

It is important to distinguish between biomedical and behavioral research, on the one hand, and the practice of accepted therapy on the other, in order to know what activities ought to undergo review for the protection of human subjects of research. The distinction between research and practice is blurred partly because both often occur together (as in research designed to evaluate a therapy) and partly because notable departures from standard practice are often called "experimental" when "research" are not carefully defined.

For the most part, the term "practice" refers to interventions that are designed solely to enhance the well-being of an individual patient or client and that have a reasonable expectation of success. The purpose of medical or behavioral practice is to provide diagnosis, preventive treatment or therapy to particular individuals.[2] By contrast, the term "research' designates an activity designed to test an hypothesis, permit conclusions to be drawn, and thereby to develop or contribute to generalizable knowledge (expressed, for example, in theories, principles, and statements of relationships). Research is usually described in a formal protocol that sets forth an objective and a set of procedures designed to reach that objective.

When a clinician departs in a significant way from standard or accepted practice, the innovation does not, in and of itself, constitute research. The fact that a procedure is "experimental," in the sense of new, untested or different, does not automatically place it in the category of research. Radically new procedures of this description should, however, be made the object of formal research at an early stage in order to determine whether they are safe and effective. Thus, it is the responsibility of medical practice committees, for example, to insist that a major innovation be incorporated into a formal research project.[3]

Research and practice may be carried on together when research is designed to evaluate the safety and efficacy of a therapy. This need not cause any confusion regarding whether or not the activity requires review; the general rule is that if there is any element of research in an activity, that activity should undergo review for the protection of human subjects.

Part B: Basic Ethical Principles

B. Basic Ethical Principles

The expression "basic ethical principles" refers to those general judgments that serve as a basic justification for the many particular ethical prescriptions and evaluations of human actions. Three basic principles, among those generally accepted in our cultural tradition, are particularly relevant to the ethics of research involving human subjects: the principles of respect of persons, beneficence and justice.

1. Respect for Persons. — Respect for persons incorporates at least two ethical convictions: first, that individuals should be treated as autonomous agents, and second, that persons with diminished autonomy are entitled to protection. The principle of respect for persons thus divides into two separate moral requirements: the requirement to acknowledge autonomy and the requirement to protect those with diminished autonomy.

An autonomous person is an individual capable of deliberation about personal goals and of acting under the direction of such deliberation. To respect autonomy is to give weight to autonomous persons' considered opinions and choices while refraining from obstructing their actions unless they are clearly detrimental to others. To show lack of respect for an autonomous agent is to repudiate that person's considered judgments, to deny an individual the freedom to act on those considered judgments, or to withhold information necessary to make a considered judgment, when there are no compelling reasons to do so.

However, not every human being is capable of self-determination. The capacity for self-determination matures during an individual's life, and some individuals lose this capacity wholly or in part because of illness, mental disability, or circumstances that severely restrict liberty. Respect for the immature and the incapacitated may require protecting them as they mature or while they are incapacitated.

Some persons are in need of extensive protection, even to the point of excluding them from activities which may harm them; other persons require little protection beyond making sure they undertake activities freely and with awareness of possible adverse consequence. The extent of protection afforded should depend upon the risk of harm and the likelihood of benefit. The judgment that any individual lacks autonomy should be periodically reevaluated and will vary in different situations.

In most cases of research involving human subjects, respect for persons demands that subjects enter into the research voluntarily and with adequate information. In some situations, however, application of the principle is not obvious. The involvement of prisoners as subjects of research provides an instructive example. On the one hand, it would seem that the principle of respect for persons requires that prisoners not be deprived of the opportunity to volunteer for research. On the other hand, under prison conditions they may be subtly coerced or unduly influenced to engage in research activities for which they would not otherwise volunteer. Respect for persons would then dictate that prisoners be protected. Whether to allow prisoners to "volunteer" or to "protect" them presents a dilemma. Respecting persons, in most hard cases, is often a matter of balancing competing claims urged by the principle of respect itself.

2. Beneficence. — Persons are treated in an ethical manner not only by respecting their decisions and protecting them from harm, but also by making efforts to secure their well-being. Such treatment falls under the principle of beneficence. The term "beneficence" is often understood to cover acts of kindness or charity that go beyond strict obligation. In this document, beneficence is understood in a stronger sense, as an obligation. Two general rules have been formulated as complementary expressions of beneficent actions in this sense: (1) do not harm and (2) maximize possible benefits and minimize possible harms.

The Hippocratic maxim "do no harm" has long been a fundamental principle of medical ethics. Claude Bernard extended it to the realm of research, saying that one should not injure one person regardless of the benefits that might come to others. However, even avoiding harm requires learning what is harmful; and, in the process of obtaining this information, persons may be exposed to risk of harm. Further, the Hippocratic Oath requires physicians to benefit their patients "according to their best judgment." Learning what will in fact benefit may require exposing persons to risk. The problem posed by these imperatives is to decide when it is justifiable to seek certain benefits despite the risks involved, and when the benefits should be foregone because of the risks.

The obligations of beneficence affect both individual investigators and society at large, because they extend both to particular research projects and to the entire enterprise of research. In the case of particular projects, investigators and members of their institutions are obliged to give forethought to the maximization of benefits and the reduction of risk that might occur from the research investigation. In the case of scientific research in general, members of the larger society are obliged to recognize the longer term benefits and risks that may result from the improvement of knowledge and from the development of novel medical, psychotherapeutic, and social procedures.

The principle of beneficence often occupies a well-defined justifying role in many areas of research involving human subjects. An example is found in research involving children. Effective ways of treating childhood diseases and fostering healthy development are benefits that serve to justify research involving children — even when individual research subjects are not direct beneficiaries. Research also makes it possible to avoid the harm that may result from the application of previously accepted routine practices that on closer investigation turn out to be dangerous. But the role of the principle of beneficence is not always so unambiguous. A difficult ethical problem remains, for example, about research that presents more than minimal risk without immediate prospect of direct benefit to the children involved. Some have argued that such research is inadmissible, while others have pointed out that this limit would rule out much research promising great benefit to children in the future. Here again, as with all hard cases, the different claims covered by the principle of beneficence may come into conflict and force difficult choices.

3. Justice. — Who ought to receive the benefits of research and bear its burdens? This is a question of justice, in the sense of "fairness in distribution" or "what is deserved." An injustice occurs when some benefit to which a person is entitled is denied without good reason or when some burden is imposed unduly. Another way of conceiving the principle of justice is that equals ought to be treated equally. However, this statement requires explication. Who is equal and who is unequal? What considerations justify departure from equal distribution? Almost all commentators allow that distinctions based on experience, age, deprivation, competence, merit and position do sometimes constitute criteria justifying differential treatment for certain purposes. It is necessary, then, to explain in what respects people should be treated equally. There are several widely accepted formulations of just ways to distribute burdens and benefits. Each formulation mentions some relevant property on the basis of which burdens and benefits should be distributed. These formulations are (1) to each person an equal share, (2) to each person according to individual need, (3) to each person according to individual effort, (4) to each person according to societal contribution, and (5) to each person according to merit.

Questions of justice have long been associated with social practices such as punishment, taxation and political representation. Until recently these questions have not generally been associated with scientific research. However, they are foreshadowed even in the earliest reflections on the ethics of research involving human subjects. For example, during the 19th and early 20th centuries the burdens of serving as research subjects fell largely upon poor ward patients, while the benefits of improved medical care flowed primarily to private patients. Subsequently, the exploitation of unwilling prisoners as research subjects in Nazi concentration camps was condemned as a particularly flagrant injustice. In this country, in the 1940's, the Tuskegee syphilis study used disadvantaged, rural black men to study the untreated course of a disease that is by no means confined to that population. These subjects were deprived of demonstrably effective treatment in order not to interrupt the project, long after such treatment became generally available.

Against this historical background, it can be seen how conceptions of justice are relevant to research involving human subjects. For example, the selection of research subjects needs to be scrutinized in order to determine whether some classes (e.g., welfare patients, particular racial and ethnic minorities, or persons confined to institutions) are being systematically selected simply because of their easy availability, their compromised position, or their manipulability, rather than for reasons directly related to the problem being studied. Finally, whenever research supported by public funds leads to the development of therapeutic devices and procedures, justice demands both that these not provide advantages only to those who can afford them and that such research should not unduly involve persons from groups unlikely to be among the beneficiaries of subsequent applications of the research.

Part C: Applications

C. Applications

Applications of the general principles to the conduct of research leads to consideration of the following requirements: informed consent, risk/benefit assessment, and the selection of subjects of research.

1. Informed Consent. — Respect for persons requires that subjects, to the degree that they are capable, be given the opportunity to choose what shall or shall not happen to them. This opportunity is provided when adequate standards for informed consent are satisfied.

While the importance of informed consent is unquestioned, controversy prevails over the nature and possibility of an informed consent.

Nonetheless, there is widespread agreement that the consent process can be analyzed as containing three elements: information, comprehension and voluntariness.

Information. Most codes of research establish specific items for disclosure intended to assure that subjects are given sufficient information. These items generally include: the research procedure, their purposes, risks and anticipated benefits, alternative procedures (where therapy is involved), and a statement offering the subject the opportunity to ask questions and to withdraw at any time from the research. Additional items have been proposed, including how subjects are selected, the person responsible for the research, etc.

However, a simple listing of items does not answer the question of what the standard should be for judging how much and what sort of information should be provided. One standard frequently invoked in medical practice, namely the information commonly provided by practitioners in the field or in the locale, is inadequate since research takes place precisely when a common understanding does not exist. Another standard, currently popular in malpractice law, requires the practitioner to reveal the information that reasonable persons would wish to know in order to make a decision regarding their care. This, too, seems insufficient since the research subject, being in essence a volunteer, may wish to know considerably more about risks gratuitously undertaken than do patients who deliver themselves into the hand of a clinician for needed care. It may be that a standard of "the reasonable volunteer" should be proposed: the extent and nature of information should be such that persons, knowing that the procedure is neither necessary for their care nor perhaps fully understood, can decide whether they wish to participate in the furthering of knowledge. Even when some direct benefit to them is anticipated, the subjects should understand clearly the range of risk and the voluntary nature of participation.

A special problem of consent arises where informing subjects of some pertinent aspect of the research is likely to impair the validity of the research. In many cases, it is sufficient to indicate to subjects that they are being invited to participate in research of which some features will not be revealed until the research is concluded. In all cases of research involving incomplete disclosure, such research is justified only if it is clear that (1) incomplete disclosure is truly necessary to accomplish the goals of the research, (2) there are no undisclosed risks to subjects that are more than minimal, and (3) there is an adequate plan for debriefing subjects, when appropriate, and for dissemination of research results to them. Information about risks should never be withheld for the purpose of eliciting the cooperation of subjects, and truthful answers should always be given to direct questions about the research. Care should be taken to distinguish cases in which disclosure would destroy or invalidate the research from cases in which disclosure would simply inconvenience the investigator.

Comprehension. The manner and context in which information is conveyed is as important as the information itself. For example, presenting information in a disorganized and rapid fashion, allowing too little time for consideration or curtailing opportunities for questioning, all may adversely affect a subject's ability to make an informed choice.

Because the subject's ability to understand is a function of intelligence, rationality, maturity and language, it is necessary to adapt the presentation of the information to the subject's capacities. Investigators are responsible for ascertaining that the subject has comprehended the information. While there is always an obligation to ascertain that the information about risk to subjects is complete and adequately comprehended, when the risks are more serious, that obligation increases. On occasion, it may be suitable to give some oral or written tests of comprehension.

Special provision may need to be made when comprehension is severely limited — for example, by conditions of immaturity or mental disability. Each class of subjects that one might consider as incompetent (e.g., infants and young children, mentally disable patients, the terminally ill and the comatose) should be considered on its own terms. Even for these persons, however, respect requires giving them the opportunity to choose to the extent they are able, whether or not to participate in research. The objections of these subjects to involvement should be honored, unless the research entails providing them a therapy unavailable elsewhere. Respect for persons also requires seeking the permission of other parties in order to protect the subjects from harm. Such persons are thus respected both by acknowledging their own wishes and by the use of third parties to protect them from harm.

The third parties chosen should be those who are most likely to understand the incompetent subject's situation and to act in that person's best interest. The person authorized to act on behalf of the subject should be given an opportunity to observe the research as it proceeds in order to be able to withdraw the subject from the research, if such action appears in the subject's best interest.

Voluntariness. An agreement to participate in research constitutes a valid consent only if voluntarily given. This element of informed consent requires conditions free of coercion and undue influence. Coercion occurs when an overt threat of harm is intentionally presented by one person to another in order to obtain compliance. Undue influence, by contrast, occurs through an offer of an excessive, unwarranted, inappropriate or improper reward or other overture in order to obtain compliance. Also, inducements that would ordinarily be acceptable may become undue influences if the subject is especially vulnerable.

Unjustifiable pressures usually occur when persons in positions of authority or commanding influence — especially where possible sanctions are involved — urge a course of action for a subject. A continuum of such influencing factors exists, however, and it is impossible to state precisely where justifiable persuasion ends and undue influence begins. But undue influence would include actions such as manipulating a person's choice through the controlling influence of a close relative and threatening to withdraw health services to which an individual would otherwise be entitle.

2. Assessment of Risks and Benefits. — The assessment of risks and benefits requires a careful arrayal of relevant data, including, in some cases, alternative ways of obtaining the benefits sought in the research. Thus, the assessment presents both an opportunity and a responsibility to gather systematic and comprehensive information about proposed research. For the investigator, it is a means to examine whether the proposed research is properly designed. For a review committee, it is a method for determining whether the risks that will be presented to subjects are justified. For prospective subjects, the assessment will assist the determination whether or not to participate.

The Nature and Scope of Risks and Benefits. The requirement that research be justified on the basis of a favorable risk/benefit assessment bears a close relation to the principle of beneficence, just as the moral requirement that informed consent be obtained is derived primarily from the principle of respect for persons. The term "risk" refers to a possibility that harm may occur. However, when expressions such as "small risk" or "high risk" are used, they usually refer (often ambiguously) both to the chance (probability) of experiencing a harm and the severity (magnitude) of the envisioned harm.

The term "benefit" is used in the research context to refer to something of positive value related to health or welfare. Unlike, "risk," "benefit" is not a term that expresses probabilities. Risk is properly contrasted to probability of benefits, and benefits are properly contrasted with harms rather than risks of harm. Accordingly, so-called risk/benefit assessments are concerned with the probabilities and magnitudes of possible harm and anticipated benefits. Many kinds of possible harms and benefits need to be taken into account. There are, for example, risks of psychological harm, physical harm, legal harm, social harm and economic harm and the corresponding benefits. While the most likely types of harms to research subjects are those of psychological or physical pain or injury, other possible kinds should not be overlooked.

Risks and benefits of research may affect the individual subjects, the families of the individual subjects, and society at large (or special groups of subjects in society). Previous codes and Federal regulations have required that risks to subjects be outweighed by the sum of both the anticipated benefit to the subject, if any, and the anticipated benefit to society in the form of knowledge to be gained from the research. In balancing these different elements, the risks and benefits affecting the immediate research subject will normally carry special weight. On the other hand, interests other than those of the subject may on some occasions be sufficient by themselves to justify the risks involved in the research, so long as the subjects' rights have been protected. Beneficence thus requires that we protect against risk of harm to subjects and also that we be concerned about the loss of the substantial benefits that might be gained from research.

The Systematic Assessment of Risks and Benefits. It is commonly said that benefits and risks must be "balanced" and shown to be "in a favorable ratio." The metaphorical character of these terms draws attention to the difficulty of making precise judgments. Only on rare occasions will quantitative techniques be available for the scrutiny of research protocols. However, the idea of systematic, nonarbitrary analysis of risks and benefits should be emulated insofar as possible. This ideal requires those making decisions about the justifiability of research to be thorough in the accumulation and assessment of information about all aspects of the research, and to consider alternatives systematically. This procedure renders the assessment of research more rigorous and precise, while making communication between review board members and investigators less subject to misinterpretation, misinformation and conflicting judgments. Thus, there should first be a determination of the validity of the presuppositions of the research; then the nature, probability and magnitude of risk should be distinguished with as much clarity as possible. The method of ascertaining risks should be explicit, especially where there is no alternative to the use of such vague categories as small or slight risk. It should also be determined whether an investigator's estimates of the probability of harm or benefits are reasonable, as judged by known facts or other available studies.

Finally, assessment of the justifiability of research should reflect at least the following considerations: (i) Brutal or inhumane treatment of human subjects is never morally justified. (ii) Risks should be reduced to those necessary to achieve the research objective. It should be determined whether it is in fact necessary to use human subjects at all. Risk can perhaps never be entirely eliminated, but it can often be reduced by careful attention to alternative procedures. (iii) When research involves significant risk of serious impairment, review committees should be extraordinarily insistent on the justification of the risk (looking usually to the likelihood of benefit to the subject — or, in some rare cases, to the manifest voluntariness of the participation). (iv) When vulnerable populations are involved in research, the appropriateness of involving them should itself be demonstrated. A number of variables go into such judgments, including the nature and degree of risk, the condition of the particular population involved, and the nature and level of the anticipated benefits. (v) Relevant risks and benefits must be thoroughly arrayed in documents and procedures used in the informed consent process.

3. Selection of Subjects. — Just as the principle of respect for persons finds expression in the requirements for consent, and the principle of beneficence in risk/benefit assessment, the principle of justice gives rise to moral requirements that there be fair procedures and outcomes in the selection of research subjects.

Justice is relevant to the selection of subjects of research at two levels: the social and the individual. Individual justice in the selection of subjects would require that researchers exhibit fairness: thus, they should not offer potentially beneficial research only to some patients who are in their favor or select only "undesirable" persons for risky research. Social justice requires that distinction be drawn between classes of subjects that ought, and ought not, to participate in any particular kind of research, based on the ability of members of that class to bear burdens and on the appropriateness of placing further burdens on already burdened persons. Thus, it can be considered a matter of social justice that there is an order of preference in the selection of classes of subjects (e.g., adults before children) and that some classes of potential subjects (e.g., the institutionalized mentally infirm or prisoners) may be involved as research subjects, if at all, only on certain conditions.

Injustice may appear in the selection of subjects, even if individual subjects are selected fairly by investigators and treated fairly in the course of research. Thus injustice arises from social, racial, sexual and cultural biases institutionalized in society. Thus, even if individual researchers are treating their research subjects fairly, and even if IRBs are taking care to assure that subjects are selected fairly within a particular institution, unjust social patterns may nevertheless appear in the overall distribution of the burdens and benefits of research. Although individual institutions or investigators may not be able to resolve a problem that is pervasive in their social setting, they can consider distributive justice in selecting research subjects.

Some populations, especially institutionalized ones, are already burdened in many ways by their infirmities and environments. When research is proposed that involves risks and does not include a therapeutic component, other less burdened classes of persons should be called upon first to accept these risks of research, except where the research is directly related to the specific conditions of the class involved. Also, even though public funds for research may often flow in the same directions as public funds for health care, it seems unfair that populations dependent on public health care constitute a pool of preferred research subjects if more advantaged populations are likely to be the recipients of the benefits.

One special instance of injustice results from the involvement of vulnerable subjects. Certain groups, such as racial minorities, the economically disadvantaged, the very sick, and the institutionalized may continually be sought as research subjects, owing to their ready availability in settings where research is conducted. Given their dependent status and their frequently compromised capacity for free consent, they should be protected against the danger of being involved in research solely for administrative convenience, or because they are easy to manipulate as a result of their illness or socioeconomic condition.

---

[1] Since 1945, various codes for the proper and responsible conduct of human experimentation in medical research have been adopted by different organizations. The best known of these codes are the Nuremberg Code of 1947, the Helsinki Declaration of 1964 (revised in 1975), and the 1971 Guidelines (codified into Federal Regulations in 1974) issued by the U.S. Department of Health, Education, and Welfare Codes for the conduct of social and behavioral research have also been adopted, the best known being that of the American Psychological Association, published in 1973.

[2] Although practice usually involves interventions designed solely to enhance the well-being of a particular individual, interventions are sometimes applied to one individual for the enhancement of the well-being of another (e.g., blood donation, skin grafts, organ transplants) or an intervention may have the dual purpose of enhancing the well-being of a particular individual, and, at the same time, providing some benefit to others (e.g., vaccination, which protects both the person who is vaccinated and society generally). The fact that some

forms of practice have elements other than immediate benefit to the individual receiving an intervention, however, should not confuse the general distinction between research and practice. Even when a procedure applied in practice may benefit some other person, it remains an intervention designed to enhance the well-being of a particular individual or groups of individuals; thus, it is practice and need not be reviewed as research.

[3] Because the problems related to social experimentation may differ substantially from those of biomedical and behavioral research, the Commission specifically declines to make any policy determination regarding such research at this time. Rather, the Commission believes that the problem ought to be addressed by one of its successor bodies.

CODE OF FEDERAL REGULATIONS

Title 21 - Food and Drugs

Chapter I - Food and Drug Administration,
Department of Health and Human Services

Part 50 - Protection of Human Subjects

Part 56 - Institutional Review Boards

Part 312- Investigational New Drug Application

Part 600- Biological Products

Part 812- Investigational Device Exemptions

Title 45 - Public Welfare

Office for Protection from Research Risks
Department of Health and Human Services

Part 46 - Protection of Human Subjects

Note: These regulations were issued in April of 1999. These regulations
are subject to periodic revisions.

PART 50—PROTECTION OF HUMAN SUBJECTS

Subpart A—General Provisions

Sec. 50.1 Scope.

(a) This part applies to all clinical investigations regulated by the Food and Drug Administration under sections 505(i), 507(d), and 520(g) of the Federal Food, Drug, and Cosmetic Act, as well as clinical investigations that support applications for research or marketing permits for products regulated by the Food and Drug Administration, including food and color additives, drugs for human use, medical devices for human use, biological products for human use, and electronic products. Additional specific obligations and commitments of, and standards of conduct for, persons who sponsor or monitor clinical investigations involving particular test articles may also be found in other parts (e.g., parts 312 and 812). Compliance with these parts is intended to protect the rights and safety of subjects involved in investigations filed with the Food and Drug Administration pursuant to sections 406, 409, 502, 503, 505, 506, 507, 510, 513-516, 518-520, 721, and 801 of the Federal Food, Drug, and Cosmetic Act and sections 351 and 354-360F of the Public Health Service Act.

(b) References in this part to regulatory sections of the Code of Federal Regulations are to chapter I of title 21, unless otherwise noted.

[45 FR 36390, May 30, 1980; 46 FR 8979, Jan. 27, 1981]

Sec. 50.3 Definitions.

As used in this part:

(a) Act means the Federal Food, Drug, and Cosmetic Act, as amended (secs. 201—902, 52 Stat. 1040 et seq. as amended (21 U.S.C. 321—392)).

(b) Application for research or marketing permit includes:

(1) A color additive petition, described in part 71.

(2) A food additive petition, described in parts 171 and 571.

(3) Data and information about a substance submitted as part of the procedures for establishing that the substance is generally recognized as safe for use that results or may reasonably be expected to result, directly or indirectly, in its becoming a component or otherwise affecting the characteristics of any food, described in Secs. 170.30 and 570.30.

(4) Data and information about a food additive submitted as part of the procedures for food additives permitted to be used on an interim basis pending additional study, described in Sec. 180.1.

(5) Data and information about a substance submitted as part of the procedures for establishing a tolerance for unavoidable contaminants in food and food-packaging materials, described in section 406 of the act.

(6) An investigational new drug application, described in part 312 of this chapter.

(7) A new drug application, described in part 314.

(8) Data and information about the bioavailability or bioequivalence of drugs for human use submitted as part of the procedures for issuing, amending, or repealing a bioequivalence requirement, described in part 320.

(9) Data and information about an over-the-counter drug for human use submitted as part of the procedures for classifying these drugs as generally recognized as safe and effective and not misbranded, described in part 330.

(10) Data and information about a prescription drug for human use submitted as part of the procedures for classifying these drugs as generally recognized as safe and effective and not misbranded, described in this chapter.

(11) Data and information about an antibiotic drug submitted as part of the procedures for issuing, amending, or repealing regulations for these drugs, described in Sec. 314.300 of this chapter.

(12) An application for a biological product license, described in part 601.

(13) Data and information about a biological product submitted as part of the procedures for determining that licensed biological products are safe and effective and not misbranded, described in part 601.

(14) Data and information about an in vitro diagnostic product submitted as part of the procedures for establishing, amending, or repealing a standard for these products, described in part 809.

(15) An Application for an Investigational Device Exemption, described in part 812.

(16) Data and information about a medical device submitted as part of the procedures for classifying these devices, described in section 513.

(17) Data and information about a medical device submitted as part of the procedures for establishing, amending, or repealing a standard for these devices, described in section 514.

(18) An application for premarket approval of a medical device, described in section 515.

(19) A product development protocol for a medical device, described in section 515.

(20) Data and information about an electronic product submitted as part of the procedures for establishing, amending, or repealing a standard for these products, described in section 358 of the Public Health Service Act.

(21) Data and information about an electronic product submitted as part of the procedures for obtaining a variance from any electronic product performance standard, as described in Sec. 1010.4.

(22) Data and information about an electronic product submitted as part of the procedures for granting, amending, or extending an exemption from a radiation safety performance standard, as described in Sec. 1010.5.

(c) Clinical investigation means any experiment that involves a test article and one or more human subjects and that either is subject to requirements for prior submission to the Food and Drug Administration under section 505(i), 507(d), or 520(g) of the act, or is not subject to requirements for prior submission to the Food and Drug Administration under these sections of the act, but the results of which are intended to be submitted later to, or held for inspection by, the Food and Drug Administration as part of an application for a research or marketing permit. The term does not include experiments that are subject to the provisions of part 58 of this chapter, regarding nonclinical laboratory studies.

(d) Investigator means an individual who actually conducts a clinical investigation, i.e., under whose immediate direction the test article is administered or dispensed to, or used involving, a subject, or, in the event of an investigation conducted by a team of individuals, is the responsible leader of that team.

(e) Sponsor means a person who initiates a clinical investigation, but who does not actually conduct the investigation, i.e., the test article is administered or dispensed to or used involving, a subject under the immediate direction of another individual. A person other than an individual (e.g., corporation or agency) that uses one or more of its own employees to conduct a clinical investigation it has initiated is considered to be a sponsor (not a sponsor-investigator), and the employees are considered to be investigators.

(f) Sponsor-investigator means an individual who both initiates and actually conducts, alone or with others, a clinical investigation, i.e., under whose immediate direction the test article is administered or dispensed to, or used involving, a subject. The term does not include any person other than an individual, e.g., corporation or agency.

(g) Human subject means an individual who is or becomes a participant in research, either as a recipient of the test article or as a control. A subject may be either a healthy human or a patient.

(h) Institution means any public or private entity or agency (including Federal, State, and other agencies). The word facility as used in section 520(g) of the act is deemed to be synonymous with the term institution for purposes of this part.

(i) Institutional review board (IRB) means any board, committee, or other group formally designated by an institution to review biomedical research involving humans as subjects, to approve the initiation of and conduct periodic review of such research. The term has the same meaning as the phrase institutional review committee as used in section 520(g) of the act.

(j) Test article means any drug (including a biological product for human use), medical device for human use, human food additive, color additive, electronic product, or any other article subject to regulation under the act or under sections 351 and 354-360F of the Public Health Service Act (42 U.S.C. 262 and 263b-263n).

(k) Minimal risk means that the probability and magnitude of harm or discomfort anticipated in the research are not greater in and of themselves than those ordinarily encountered in daily life or during the performance of routine physical or psychological examinations or tests.

(l) Legally authorized representative means an individual or judicial or other body authorized under applicable law to consent on behalf of a prospective subject to the subject's participation in the procedure(s) involved in the research.

(m) Family member means any one of the following legally competent persons: Spouse; parents; children (including adopted children); brothers, sisters, and spouses of brothers and sisters; and any individual related by blood or affinity whose close association with the subject is the equivalent of a family relationship.

[45 FR 36390, May 30, 1980, as amended at 46 FR 8950, Jan. 27, 1981; 54 FR 9038, Mar. 3, 1989; 56 FR 28028, June 18, 1991; 61 FR 51528, Oct. 2, 1996; 62 FR 39440, July 23, 1997]

Subpart B—Informed Consent of Human Subjects

Sec. 50.20 General requirements for informed consent.

Source: 46 FR 8951, Jan. 27, 1981, unless otherwise noted.

Except as provided in Sec. 50.23, no investigator may involve a human being as a subject in research covered by these regulations unless the investigator has obtained the legally effective informed consent of the subject or the subject's legally authorized representative. An investigator shall seek such consent only under circumstances that provide the prospective subject or the representative sufficient opportunity to consider whether or not to participate and that minimize the possibility of coercion or undue influence. The information that is given to the subject or the representative shall be in language understandable to the subject or the representative. No informed consent, whether oral or written, may include any exculpatory language through which the subject or the representative is made to waive or appear to waive any of the subject's legal rights, or releases or appears to release the investigator, the sponsor, the institution, or its agents from liability for negligence.

Sec. 50.23 Exception from general requirements.

(a) The obtaining of informed consent shall be deemed feasible unless, before use of the test article (except as provided in paragraph (b) of this section), both the investigator and a physician who is not otherwise participating in the clinical investigation certify in writing all of the following:

(1) The human subject is confronted by a life-threatening situation necessitating the use of the test article.

(2) Informed consent cannot be obtained from the subject because of an inability to communicate with, or obtain legally effective consent from, the subject.

(3) Time is not sufficient to obtain consent from the subject's legal representative.

(4) There is available no alternative method of approved or generally recognized therapy that provides an equal or greater likelihood of saving the life of the subject.

(b) If immediate use of the test article is, in the investigator's opinion, required to preserve the life of the subject, and time is not sufficient to obtain the independent determination required in paragraph (a) of this section in advance of using the test article, the determinations of the clinical investigator shall be made and, within 5 working days after the use of the article, be reviewed and evaluated in writing by a physician who is not participating in the clinical investigation.

(c) The documentation required in paragraph (a) or (b) of this section shall be submitted to the IRB within 5 working days after the use of the test article.

(d)(1) The Commissioner may also determine that obtaining informed consent is not feasible when the Assistant Secretary of Defense (Health Affairs) requests such a determination in connection with the use of an investigational drug (including an antibiotic or biological product) in a specific protocol under an investigational new drug application (IND) sponsored by the Department of Defense (DOD). DOD's request for a determination that obtaining informed consent from military personnel is not feasible must be limited to a specific military operation involving combat or the immediate threat of combat. The request must also include a written justification supporting the conclusions of the physician(s) responsible for the medical care of the military personnel involved and the investigator(s) identified in the IND that a military combat exigency exists because of special military combat (actual or threatened) circumstances in which, in order to facilitate the accomplishment of the military mission, preservation of the health of the individual and the safety of other personnel require that a particular treatment be provided to a specified group of military personnel, without regard to what might be any individual's personal preference for no treatment or for some alternative treatment. The written request must also include a statement that a duly constituted institutional review board has reviewed and approved the use of the investigational drug without informed consent. The Commissioner may find that informed consent is not feasible only when withholding treatment would be contrary to the best interests of military personnel and there is no available satisfactory alternative therapy.

(2) In reaching a determination under paragraph (d)(1) of this section that obtaining informed consent is not feasible and withholding treatment would be contrary to the best interests of military personnel, the Commissioner will review the request submitted under paragraph (d)(1) of this section and take into account all pertinent factors, including, but not limited to:

(i) The extent and strength of the evidence of the safety and effectiveness of the investigational drug for the intended use;

(ii) The context in which the drug will be administered, e.g., whether it is intended for use in a battlefield or hospital setting or whether it will be self-administered or will be administered by a health professional;

(iii) The nature of the disease or condition for which the preventive or therapeutic treatment is intended; and

(iv) The nature of the information to be provided to the recipients of the drug concerning the potential benefits and risks of taking or not taking the drug.

(3) The Commissioner may request a recommendation from appropriate experts before reaching a determination on a request submitted under paragraph (d)(1) of this section.

(4) A determination by the Commissioner that obtaining informed consent is not feasible and withholding treatment would be contrary to the best interests of military personnel will expire at the end of 1 year, unless renewed at DOD's request, or when DOD informs the Commissioner that the specific military operation creating the need for the use of the investigational drug has ended, whichever is earlier. The Commissioner may also revoke this determination based on changed circumstances.

[46 FR 8951, Jan. 27, 1981, as amended at 55 FR 52817, Dec. 21, 1990]

Sec. 50.24 Exception from informed consent requirements for emergency research.

(a) The IRB responsible for the review, approval, and continuing review of the clinical investigation described in this section may approve that investigation without requiring that informed consent of all research subjects be obtained if the IRB (with the concurrence of a licensed physician who is a member of or consultant to the IRB and who is not otherwise participating in the clinical investigation) finds and documents each of the following:

(1) The human subjects are in a life-threatening situation, available treatments are unproven or unsatisfactory, and the collection of valid scientific evidence, which may include evidence obtained through randomized placebo-controlled investigations, is necessary to determine the safety and effectiveness of particular interventions.

(2) Obtaining informed consent is not feasible because:

(i) The subjects will not be able to give their informed consent as a result of their medical condition;

(ii) The intervention under investigation must be administered before consent from the subjects' legally authorized representatives is feasible; and

(iii) There is no reasonable way to identify prospectively the individuals likely to become eligible for participation in the clinical investigation.

(3) Participation in the research holds out the prospect of direct benefit to the subjects because:

(i) Subjects are facing a life-threatening situation that necessitates intervention;

(ii) Appropriate animal and other preclinical studies have been conducted, and the information derived from those studies and related evidence support the potential for the intervention to provide a direct benefit to the individual subjects; and

(iii) Risks associated with the investigation are reasonable in relation to what is known about the medical condition of the potential class of subjects, the risks and benefits of standard therapy, if any, and what is known about the risks and benefits of the proposed intervention or activity.

(4) The clinical investigation could not practicably be carried out without the waiver.

(5) The proposed investigational plan defines the length of the potential therapeutic window based on scientific evidence, and the investigator has committed to attempting to contact a legally authorized representative for each subject within that window of time and, if feasible, to asking the legally authorized representative contacted for consent within that window rather than proceeding without consent. The investigator will summarize efforts made to contact legally authorized representatives and make this information available to the IRB at the time of continuing review.

(6) The IRB has reviewed and approved informed consent procedures and an informed consent document consistent with Sec. 50.25. These procedures and the informed consent document are to be used with subjects or their legally authorized representatives in situations where use of such procedures and documents is feasible. The IRB has reviewed and approved procedures and information to be used when providing an opportunity for a family member to object to a subject's participation in the clinical investigation consistent with paragraph (a)(7)(v) of this section.

(7) Additional protections of the rights and welfare of the subjects will be provided, including, at least:

(i) Consultation (including, where appropriate, consultation carried out by the IRB) with representatives of the communities in which the clinical investigation will be conducted and from which the subjects will be drawn;

(ii) Public disclosure to the communities in which the clinical investigation will be conducted and from which the subjects will be drawn, prior to initiation of the clinical investigation, of plans for the investigation and its risks and expected benefits;

(iii) Public disclosure of sufficient information following completion of the clinical investigation to apprise the community and researchers of the study, including the demographic characteristics of the research population, and its results;

(iv) Establishment of an independent data monitoring committee to exercise oversight of the clinical investigation; and

(v) If obtaining informed consent is not feasible and a legally authorized representative is not reasonably available, the investigator has committed, if feasible, to attempting to contact within the therapeutic window the subject's family member who is not a legally authorized representative, and asking whether he or she objects to the subject's participation in the clinical investigation. The investigator will summarize efforts made to contact family members and make this information available to the IRB at the time of continuing review.

(b) The IRB is responsible for ensuring that procedures are in place to inform, at the earliest feasible opportunity, each subject, or if the subject remains incapacitated, a legally authorized representative of the subject, or if such a representative is not reasonably available, a family member, of the subject's inclusion in the clinical investigation, the details of the investigation and other information contained in the informed consent document. The IRB shall also ensure that there is a procedure to inform the subject, or if the subject remains incapacitated, a legally authorized representative of the subject, or if such a representative is not reasonably available, a family member, that he or she may discontinue the subject's participation at any time without penalty or loss of benefits to which the subject is otherwise entitled. If a legally authorized representative or family member is told about the clinical investigation and the subject's condition improves, the subject is also to be informed as soon as feasible. If a subject is entered into a clinical investigation with waived consent and the subject dies before a legally authorized representative or family member can be contacted, information about the clinical investigation is to be provided to the subject's legally authorized representative or family member, if feasible.

(c) The IRB determinations required by paragraph (a) of this section and the documentation required by paragraph (e) of this section are to be retained by the IRB for at least 3 years after completion of the clinical investigation, and the records shall be accessible for inspection and copying by FDA in accordance with Sec. 56.115(b) of this chapter.

(d) Protocols involving an exception to the informed consent requirement under this section must be performed under a separate investigational new drug application (IND) or investigational device exemption (IDE) that clearly identifies such protocols as protocols that may include subjects who are unable to consent. The submission of those protocols in a separate IND/IDE is required even if an IND for the same drug product or an IDE for the same device already exists. Applications for investigations under this section may not be submitted as amendments under Secs. 312.30 or 812.35 of this chapter.

(e) If an IRB determines that it cannot approve a clinical investigation because the investigation does not meet the criteria in the exception provided under paragraph (a) of this section or because of other relevant ethical concerns, the IRB must document its findings and provide these findings promptly in writing to the clinical investigator and to the sponsor of the clinical investigation. The sponsor of the clinical investigation must promptly disclose this information to FDA and to the sponsor's clinical investigators who are participating or are asked to participate in this or a substantially equivalent clinical investigation of the sponsor, and to other IRB's that have been, or are, asked to review this or a substantially equivalent investigation by that sponsor.

[61 FR 51528, Oct. 2, 1996]

Sec. 50.25 Elements of informed consent.

(a) Basic elements of informed consent. In seeking informed consent, the following information shall be provided to each subject:

(1) A statement that the study involves research, an explanation of the purposes of the research and the expected duration of the subject's participation, a description of the procedures to be followed, and identification of any procedures which are experimental.

(2) A description of any reasonably foreseeable risks or discomforts to the subject.

(3) A description of any benefits to the subject or to others which may reasonably be expected from the research.

(4) A disclosure of appropriate alternative procedures or courses of treatment, if any, that might be advantageous to the subject.

(5) A statement describing the extent, if any, to which confidentiality of records identifying the subject will be maintained and that notes the possibility that the Food and Drug Administration may inspect the records.

(6) For research involving more than minimal risk, an explanation as to whether any compensation and an explanation as to whether any medical treatments are available if

injury occurs and, if so, what they consist of, or where further information may be obtained.

(7) An explanation of whom to contact for answers to pertinent questions about the research and research subjects' rights, and whom to contact in the event of a research-related injury to the subject.

(8) A statement that participation is voluntary, that refusal to participate will involve no penalty or loss of benefits to which the subject is otherwise entitled, and that the subject may discontinue participation at any time without penalty or loss of benefits to which the subject is otherwise entitled.

(b) Additional elements of informed consent. When appropriate, one or more of the following elements of information shall also be provided to each subject:

(1) A statement that the particular treatment or procedure may involve risks to the subject (or to the embryo or fetus, if the subject is or may become pregnant) which are currently unforeseeable.

(2) Anticipated circumstances under which the subject's participation may be terminated by the investigator without regard to the subject's consent.

(3) Any additional costs to the subject that may result from participation in the research.

(4) The consequences of a subject's decision to withdraw from the research and procedures for orderly termination of participation by the subject.

(5) A statement that significant new findings developed during the course of the research which may relate to the subject's willingness to continue participation will be provided to the subject.

(6) The approximate number of subjects involved in the study.

(c) The informed consent requirements in these regulations are not intended to preempt any applicable Federal, State, or local laws which require additional information to be disclosed for informed consent to be legally effective.

(d) Nothing in these regulations is intended to limit the authority of a physician to provide emergency medical care to the extent the physician is permitted to do so under applicable Federal, State, or local law.

Sec. 50.27 Documentation of informed consent.

(a) Except as provided in Sec. 56.109(c), informed consent shall be documented by the use of a written consent form approved by the IRB and signed and dated by the subject or the subject's legally authorized representative at the time of consent. A copy shall be given to the person signing the form.

(b) Except as provided in Sec. 56.109(c), the consent form may be either of the following:

(1) A written consent document that embodies the elements of informed consent required by Sec. 50.25. This form may be read to the subject or the subject's legally authorized representative, but, in any event, the investigator shall give either the subject or the representative adequate opportunity to read it before it is signed.

(2) A short form written consent document stating that the elements of informed consent required by Sec. 50.25 have been presented orally to the subject or the subject's legally authorized representative. When this method is used, there shall be a witness to the oral presentation. Also, the IRB shall approve a written summary of what is to be said to the subject or the representative. Only the short form itself is to be signed by the subject or the representative. However, the witness shall sign both the short form and a copy of the summary, and the person actually obtaining the consent shall sign a copy of the summary. A copy of the summary shall be given to the subject or the representative in addition to a copy of the short form.

[46 FR 8951, Jan. 27, 1981, as amended at 61 FR 57280, Nov. 5, 1996]

PART 56—INSTITUTIONAL REVIEW BOARDS

Subpart A—General Provisions

Sec. 56.101 Scope.

(a) This part contains the general standards for the composition, operation, and responsibility of an Institutional Review Board (IRB) that reviews clinical investigations regulated by the Food and Drug Administration under sections 505(i), 507(d), and 520(g) of the act, as well as clinical investigations that support applications for research or marketing permits for products regulated by the Food and Drug Administration, including food and color additives, drugs for human use, medical devices for human use, biological products for human use, and electronic products. Compliance with this part is intended to protect the rights and welfare of human subjects involved in such investigations.

(b) References in this part to regulatory sections of the Code of Federal Regulations are to chapter I of title 21, unless otherwise noted.

Sec. 56.102 Definitions.

As used in this part:

(a) Act means the Federal Food, Drug, and Cosmetic Act, as amended (secs. 201-902, 52 Stat. 1040 et seq., as amended (21 U.S.C. 321-392)).

(b) Application for research or marketing permit includes:

(1) A color additive petition, described in part 71.

(2) Data and information regarding a substance submitted as part of the procedures for establishing that a substance is generally recognized as safe for a use which results or may reasonably be expected to result, directly or indirectly, in its becoming a component or otherwise affecting the characteristics of any food, described in Sec. 170.35.

(3) A food additive petition, described in part 171.

(4) Data and information regarding a food additive submitted as part of the procedures regarding food additives permitted to be used on an interim basis pending additional study, described in Sec. 180.1.

(5) Data and information regarding a substance submitted as part of the procedures for establishing a tolerance for unavoidable contaminants in food and food-packaging materials, described in section 406 of the act.

(6) An investigational new drug application, described in part 312 of this chapter.

(7) A new drug application, described in part 314.

(8) Data and information regarding the bioavailability or bioequivalence of drugs for human use submitted as part of the procedures for issuing, amending, or repealing a bioequivalence requirement, described in part 320.

(9) Data and information regarding an over-the-counter drug for human use submitted as part of the procedures for classifying such drugs as generally recognized as safe and effective and not misbranded, described in part 330.

(10) Data and information regarding an antibiotic drug submitted as part of the procedures for issuing, amending, or repealing regulations for such drugs, described in Sec. 314.300 of this chapter.

(11) An application for a biological product license, described in part 601.

(12) Data and information regarding a biological product submitted as part of the procedures for determining that licensed biological products are safe and effective and not misbranded, as described in part 601.

(13) An Application for an Investigational Device Exemption, described in parts 812 and 813.

(14) Data and information regarding a medical device for human use submitted as part of the procedures for classifying such devices, described in part 860.

(15) Data and information regarding a medical device for human use submitted as part of the procedures for establishing, amending, or repealing a standard for such device, described in part 861.

(16) An application for premarket approval of a medical device for human use, described in section 515 of the act.

(17) A product development protocol for a medical device for human use, described in section 515 of the act.

(18) Data and information regarding an electronic product submitted as part of the procedures for establishing, amending, or repealing a standard for such products, described in section 358 of the Public Health Service Act.

(19) Data and information regarding an electronic product submitted as part of the procedures for obtaining a variance from any electronic product performance standard, as described in Sec. 1010.4.

(20) Data and information regarding an electronic product submitted as part of the procedures for granting, amending, or extending an exemption from a radiation safety performance standard, as described in Sec. 1010.5.

(21) Data and information regarding an electronic product submitted as part of the procedures for obtaining an exemption from notification of a radiation safety defect or failure of compliance with a radiation safety performance standard, described in subpart D of part 1003.

(c) Clinical investigation means any experiment that involves a test article and one or more human subjects, and that either must meet the requirements for prior submission to the Food and Drug Administration under section 505(i), 507(d), or 520(g) of the act, or need not meet the requirements for prior submission to the Food and Drug Administration under these sections of the act, but the results of which are intended to be later submitted to, or held for inspection by, the Food and Drug Administration as part of an application for a research or marketing permit. The term does not include experiments that must meet the provisions of part 58, regarding nonclinical laboratory studies. The terms research, clinical research, clinical study, study, and clinical investigation are deemed to be synonymous for purposes of this part.

(d) Emergency use means the use of a test article on a human subject in a life-threatening situation in which no standard acceptable treatment is available, and in which there is not sufficient time to obtain IRB approval.

(e) Human subject means an individual who is or becomes a participant in research, either as a recipient of the test article or as a control. A subject may be either a healthy individual or a patient.

(f) Institution means any public or private entity or agency (including Federal, State, and other agencies). The term facility as used in section 520(g) of the act is deemed to be synonymous with the term institution for purposes of this part.

(g) Institutional Review Board (IRB) means any board, committee, or other group formally designated by an institution to review, to approve the initiation of, and to conduct periodic review of, biomedical research involving human subjects. The primary purpose of such review is to assure the protection of the rights and welfare of the human subjects. The term has the same meaning as the phrase institutional review committee as used in section 520(g) of the act.

(h) Investigator means an individual who actually conducts a clinical investigation (i.e., under whose immediate direction the test article is administered or dispensed to, or used involving, a subject) or, in the event of an investigation conducted by a team of individuals, is the responsible leader of that team.

(i) Minimal risk means that the probability and magnitude of harm or discomfort anticipated in the research are not greater in and of themselves than those ordinarily encountered in daily life or during the performance of routine physical or psychological examinations or tests.

(j) Sponsor means a person or other entity that initiates a clinical investigation, but that does not actually conduct the investigation, i.e., the test article is administered or dispensed to, or used involving, a subject under the immediate direction of another individual. A person other than an individual (e.g., a corporation or agency) that uses one or more of its own employees to conduct an investigation that it has initiated is considered to be a sponsor (not a sponsor-investigator), and the employees are considered to be investigators.

(k) Sponsor-investigator means an individual who both initiates and actually conducts, alone or with others, a clinical investigation, i.e., under whose immediate direction the test article is administered or dispensed to, or used involving, a subject. The term does not include any person other than an individual, e.g., it does not include a corporation or agency. The obligations of a sponsor-investigator under this part include both those of a sponsor and those of an investigator.

(l) Test article means any drug for human use, biological product for human use, medical device for human use, human food additive, color additive, electronic product, or any other article subject to regulation under the act or under sections 351 or 354-360F of the Public Health Service Act.

(m) IRB approval means the determination of the IRB that the clinical investigation has been reviewed and may be conducted at an institution within the constraints set forth by the IRB and by other institutional and Federal requirements.

[46 FR 8975, Jan. 27, 1981, as amended at 54 FR 9038, Mar. 3, 1989; 56 FR 28028, June 18, 1991]

Sec. 56.103 Circumstances in which IRB review is required.

(a) Except as provided in Secs. 56.104 and 56.105, any clinical investigation which must meet the requirements for prior submission (as required in parts 312, 812, and 813) to the Food and Drug Administration shall not be initiated unless that investigation has been reviewed and approved by, and remains subject to continuing review by, anIRB meeting the requirements of this part.

(b) Except as provided in Secs. 56.104 and 56.105, the Food and Drug Administration may decide not to consider in support of an application for a research or marketing permit any data or information that has been derived from a clinical investigation that has not been approved by, and that was not subject to initial and continuing review by, an IRB meeting the requirements of this part. The determination that a clinical investigation may not be considered in support of an application for a research or marketing permit does not, however, relieve the applicant for such a permit of any obligation under any other applicable regulations to submit the results of the investigation to the Food and Drug Administration.

(c) Compliance with these regulations will in no way render inapplicable pertinent Federal, State, or local laws or regulations.

[46 FR 8975, Jan. 27, 1981; 46 FR 14340, Feb. 27, 1981]

Sec. 56.104 Exemptions from IRB requirement.

The following categories of clinical investigations are exempt from the requirements of this part for IRB review:

(a) Any investigation which commenced before July 27, 1981 and was subject to requirements for IRB review under FDA regulations before that date, provided that the investigation remains subject to review of an IRB which meets the FDA requirements in effect before July 27, 1981.

(b) Any investigation commenced before July 27, 1981 and was not otherwise subject to requirements for IRB review under Food and Drug Administration regulations before that date.

(c) Emergency use of a test article, provided that such emergency use is reported to the IRB within 5 working days. Any subsequent use of the test article at the institution is subject to IRB review.

(d) Taste and food quality evaluations and consumer acceptance studies, if wholesome foods without additives are consumed or if a food is consumed that contains a food ingredient at or below the level and for a use found to be safe, or agricultural, chemical, or environmental contaminant at or below the level found to be safe, by the Food and Drug Administration or approved by the Environmental Protection Agency or the Food Safety and Inspection Service of the U.S. Department of Agriculture.

[46 FR 8975, Jan. 27, 1981, as amended at 56 FR 28028, June 18, 1991]

Sec. 56.105 Waiver of IRB requirement.

On the application of a sponsor or sponsor-investigator, the Food and Drug Administration may waive any of the requirements contained in these regulations, including the requirements for IRB review, for specific research activities or for classes of research activities, otherwise covered by these regulations.

Subpart B—Organization and Personnel

Sec. 56.107 IRB membership.

(a) Each IRB shall have at least five members, with varying backgrounds to promote complete and adequate review of research activities commonly conducted by the institution. The IRB shall be sufficiently qualified through the experience and expertise of its members, and the diversity of the members, including consideration of race, gender, cultural backgrounds, and sensitivity to such issues as community attitudes, to promote respect for its advice and counsel in safeguarding the rights and welfare of human subjects. In addition to possessing the professional competence necessary to review the specific research activities, the IRB shall be able to ascertain the acceptability of proposed research in terms of institutional commitments and regulations, applicable law, and standards or professional conduct and practice. The IRB shall therefore include persons knowledgeable in these areas. If an IRB regularly reviews research that involves a vulnerable category of subjects, such as children, prisoners, pregnant women, or handicapped or mentally disabled persons, consideration shall be given to the inclusion of one or more individuals who are knowledgeable about and experienced in working with those subjects.

(b) Every nondiscriminatory effort will be made to ensure that no IRB consists entirely of men or entirely of women, including the institution's consideration of qualified persons of both sexes, so long as no selection is made to the IRB on the basis of gender. No IRB may consist entirely of members of one profession.

(c) Each IRB shall include at least one member whose primary concerns are in the scientific area and at least one member whose primary concerns are in nonscientific areas.

(d) Each IRB shall include at least one member who is not otherwise affiliated with the institution and who is not part of the immediate family of a person who is affiliated with the institution.

(e) No IRB may have a member participate in the IRB's initial or continuing review of any project in which the member has a conflicting interest, except to provide information requested by the IRB.

(f) An IRB may, in its discretion, invite individuals with competence in special areas to assist in the review of complex issues which require expertise beyond or in addition to that available on the IRB. These individuals may not vote with the IRB.

[46 FR 8975, Jan 27, 1981, as amended at 56 FR 28028, June 18, 1991; 56 FR 29756, June 28, 1991]

Subpart C—IRB Functions and Operations

Sec. 56.108 IRB functions and operations.

In order to fulfill the requirements of these regulations, each IRB shall:

(a) Follow written procedures: (1) For conducting its initial and continuing review of research and for reporting its findings and actions to the investigator and the institution; (2) for determining which projects require review more often than annually and which projects need verification from sources other than the investigator that no material changes have occurred since previous IRB review; (3) for ensuring prompt reporting to the IRB of changes in research activity; and (4) for ensuring that changes in approved research, during the period for which IRB approval has already been given, may not be initiated without IRB review and approval except where necessary to eliminate apparent immediate hazards to the human subjects.

(b) Follow written procedures for ensuring prompt reporting to the IRB, appropriate institutional officials, and the Food and Drug Administration of: (1) Any unanticipated problems involving risks to human subjects or others; (2) any instance of serious or continuing noncompliance with these regulations or the requirements or determinations of the IRB; or (3) any suspension or termination of IRB approval.

(c) Except when an expedited review procedure is used (see Sec. 56.110), review proposed research at convened meetings at which a majority of the members of the IRB are present, including at least one member whose primary concerns are in nonscientific areas. In order for the research to be approved, it shall receive the approval of a majority of those members present at the meeting.

(Information collection requirements in this section were approved by the Office of Management and Budget (OMB) and assigned OMB control number 0910-0130)

[46 FR 8975, Jan. 27, 1981, as amended at 56 FR 28028, June 18, 1991]

Sec. 56.109 IRB review of research.

(a) An IRB shall review and have authority to approve, require modifications in (to secure approval), or disapprove all research activities covered by these regulations.

(b) An IRB shall require that information given to subjects as part of informed consent is in accordance with Sec. 50.25. The IRB may require that information, in addition to that specifically mentioned in Sec. 50.25, be given to the subjects when in the IRB's judgment the information would meaningfully add to the protection of the rights and welfare of subjects.

(c) An IRB shall require documentation of informed consent in accordance with Sec. 50.27 of this chapter, except as follows:

(1) The IRB may, for some or all subjects, waive the requirement that the subject, or the subject's legally authorized representative, sign a written consent form if it finds that the research presents no more than minimal risk of harm to subjects and involves no procedures for which written consent is normally required outside the research context; or

(2) The IRB may, for some or all subjects, find that the requirements in Sec. 50.24 of this chapter for an exception from informed consent for emergency research are met.

(d) In cases where the documentation requirement is waived under paragraph (c)(1) of this section, the IRB may require the investigator to provide subjects with a written statement regarding the research.

(e) An IRB shall notify investigators and the institution in writing of its decision to approve or disapprove the proposed research activity, or of modifications required to secure IRB approval of the research activity. If the IRB decides to disapprove a research activity, it shall include in its written notification a statement of the reasons for its decision and give the investigator an opportunity to respond in person or in writing. For investigations involving an exception to informed consent under Sec. 50.24 of this chapter, an IRB shall promptly notify in writing the investigator and the sponsor of the research when an IRB determines that it cannot approve the research because it does not meet the criteria in the exception provided under Sec. 50.24(a) of this chapter or because of other relevant ethical concerns. The written notification shall include a statement of the reasons for the IRB's determination.

(f) An IRB shall conduct continuing review of research covered by these regulations at intervals appropriate to the degree of risk, but not less than once per year, and shall have authority to observe or have a third party observe the consent process and the research.

(g) An IRB shall provide in writing to the sponsor of research involving an exception to informed consent under Sec. 50.24 of this chapter a copy of information that has been publicly disclosed under Sec. 50.24(a)(7)(ii) and (a)(7)(iii) of this chapter. The IRB shall provide this information to the sponsor promptly so that the sponsor is aware that such disclosure has occurred. Upon receipt, the sponsor shall provide copies of the information disclosed to FDA.

[46 FR 8975, Jan. 27, 1981, as amended at 61 FR 51529, Oct. 2, 1996]

Sec. 56.110 Expedited review procedures for certain kinds of research involving no more than minimal risk, and for minor changes in approved research.

(a) The Food and Drug Administration has established, and published in the Federal Register, a list of categories of research that may be reviewed by the IRB through an expedited review procedure. The list will be amended, as appropriate, through periodic republication in the Federal Register.

(b) An IRB may use the expedited review procedure to review either or both of the following: (1) Some or all of the research appearing on the list and found by the reviewer(s) to involve no more than minimal risk, (2) minor changes in previously approved research during the period (of 1 year or less) for which approval is authorized. Under an expedited review procedure, the review may be carried out by the IRB chairperson or by one or more experienced reviewers designated by the IRB chairperson from among the members of the IRB. In reviewing the research, the reviewers may exercise all of the authorities of the IRB except that the reviewers may not disapprove the research. A research activity may be disapproved only after review in accordance with the nonexpedited review procedure set forth in Sec. 56.108(c).

(c) Each IRB which uses an expedited review procedure shall adopt a method for keeping all members advised of research proposals which have been approved under the procedure.

(d) The Food and Drug Administration may restrict, suspend, or terminate an institution's or IRB's use of the expedited review procedure when necessary to protect the rights or welfare of subjects.

[46 FR 8975, Jan. 27, 1981, as amended at 56 FR 28029, June 18, 1991]

Sec. 56.111 Criteria for IRB approval of research.

(a) In order to approve research covered by these regulations the IRB shall determine that all of the following requirements are satisfied:

(1) Risks to subjects are minimized: (i) By using procedures which are consistent with sound research design and which do not unnecessarily expose subjects to risk, and (ii) whenever appropriate, by using procedures already being performed on the subjects for diagnostic or treatment purposes.

(2) Risks to subjects are reasonable in relation to anticipated benefits, if any, to subjects, and the importance of the knowledge that may be expected to result. In evaluating risks and benefits, the IRB should consider only those risks and benefits that may result from the research (as distinguished from risks and benefits of therapies that subjects would receive even if not participating in the research). The IRB should not consider possible long-range effects of applying knowledge gained in the research (for example, the possible effects of the research on public policy) as among those research risks that fall within the purview of its responsibility.

(3) Selection of subjects is equitable. In making this assessment the IRB should take into account the purposes of the research and the setting in which the research will be conducted and should be particularly cognizant of the special problems of research involving vulnerable populations, such as children, prisoners, pregnant women, handicapped, or mentally disabled persons, or economically or educationally disadvantaged persons.

(4) Informed consent will be sought from each prospective subject or the subject's legally authorized representative, in accordance with and to the extent required by part 50.

(5) Informed consent will be appropriately documented, in accordance with and to the extent required by Sec. 50.27.

(6) Where appropriate, the research plan makes adequate provision for monitoring the data collected to ensure the safety of subjects.

(7) Where appropriate, there are adequate provisions to protect the privacy of subjects and to maintain the confidentiality of data.

(b) When some or all of the subjects, such as children, prisoners, pregnant women, handicapped, or mentally disabled persons, or economically or educationally disadvantaged persons, are likely to be vulnerable to coercion or undue influence additional safeguards have been included in the study to protect the rights and welfare of these subjects.

[46 FR 8975, Jan. 27, 1981, as amended at 56 FR 28029, June 18, 1991]

PART 312—INVESTIGATIONAL NEW DRUG APPLICATION

Subpart A—General Provisions

Sec. 312.1 Scope.

(a) This part contains procedures and requirements governing the use of investigational new drugs, including procedures and requirements for the submission to, and review by, the Food and Drug Administration of investigational new drug applications (IND's). An investigational new drug for which an IND is in effect in accordance with this part is exempt from the premarketing approval requirements that are otherwise applicable and may be shipped lawfully for the purpose of conducting clinical investigations of that drug.

(b) References in this part to regulations in the Code of Federal Regulations are to chapter I of title 21, unless otherwise noted.

Sec. 312.2 Applicability.

(a) Applicability. Except as provided in this section, this part applies to all clinical investigations of products that are subject to section 505 or 507 of the Federal Food, Drug, and Cosmetic Act or to the licensing provisions of the Public Health Service Act (58 Stat. 632, as amended (42 U.S.C. 201 et seq.)).

(b) Exemptions. (1) The clinical investigation of a drug product that is lawfully marketed in the United States is exempt from the requirements of this part if all the following apply:

(i) The investigation is not intended to be reported to FDA as a well-controlled study in support of a new indication for use nor intended to be used to support any other significant change in the labeling for the drug;

(ii) If the drug that is undergoing investigation is lawfully marketed as a prescription drug product, the investigation is not intended to support a significant change in the advertising for the product;

(iii) The investigation does not involve a route of administration or dosage level or use in a patient population or other factor that significantly increases the risks (or decreases the acceptability of the risks) associated with the use of the drug product;

(iv) The investigation is conducted in compliance with the requirements for institutional review set forth in part 56 and with the requirements for informed consent set forth in part 50; and

(v) The investigation is conducted in compliance with the requirements of Sec. 312.7.

(2)(i) A clinical investigation involving an in vitro diagnostic biological product listed in paragraph (b)(2)(ii) of this section is exempt from the requirements of this part if (a) it is intended to be used in a diagnostic procedure that confirms the diagnosis made by another, medically established, diagnostic product or procedure and (b) it is shipped in compliance with Sec. 312.160.

(ii) In accordance with paragraph (b)(2)(i) of this section, the following products are exempt from the requirements of this part: (a) blood grouping serum; (b) reagent red blood cells; and (c) anti-human globulin.

(3) A drug intended solely for tests in vitro or in laboratory research animals is exempt from the requirements of this part if shipped in accordance with Sec. 312.160.

(4) FDA will not accept an application for an investigation that is exempt under the provisions of paragraph (b)(1) of this section.

(5) A clinical investigation involving use of a placebo is exempt from the requirements of this part if the investigation does not otherwise require submission of an IND.

(6) A clinical investigation involving an exception from informed consent under Sec. 50.24

of this chapter is not exempt from the requirements of this part.

(c) Bioavailability studies. The applicability of this part to in vivo bioavailability studies in humans is subject to the provisions of Sec. 320.31.

(d) Unlabeled indication. This part does not apply to the use in the practice of medicine for an unlabeled indication of a new drug or antibiotic drug product approved under part 314 or of a licensed biological product.

(e) Guidance. FDA may, on its own initiative, issue guidance on the applicability of this part to particular investigational uses of drugs. On request, FDA will advise on the applicability of this part to a planned clinical investigation.

[52 FR 8831, Mar. 19, 1987, as amended at 61 FR 51529, Oct. 2, 1996]

Sec. 312.3 Definitions and interpretations.

(a) The definitions and interpretations of terms contained in section 201 of the Act apply to those terms when used in this part:

(b) The following definitions of terms also apply to this part:

Act means the Federal Food, Drug, and Cosmetic Act (secs. 201-902, 52 Stat. 1040 et seq., as amended (21 U.S.C. 301-392)).

Clinical investigation means any experiment in which a drug is administered or dispensed to, or used involving, one or more human subjects. For the purposes of this part, an experiment is any use of a drug except for the use of a marketed drug in the course of medical practice.

Contract research organization means a person that assumes, as an independent contractor with the sponsor, one or more of the obligations of a sponsor, e.g., design of a protocol, selection or monitoring of investigations, evaluation of reports, and preparation of materials to be submitted to the Food and Drug Administration.

FDA means the Food and Drug Administration.

IND means an investigational new drug application. For purposes of this part, "IND" is synonymous with "Notice of Claimed Investigational Exemption for a New Drug."

Investigational new drug means a new drug, antibiotic drug, or biological drug that is used in a clinical investigation. The term also includes a biological product that is used in vitro for diagnostic purposes. The terms "investigational drug" and "investigational new drug" are deemed to be synonymous for purposes of this part.

Investigator means an individual who actually conducts a clinical investigation (i.e., under whose immediate direction the drug is administered or dispensed to a subject). In the event an investigation is conducted by a team of individuals, the investigator is the responsible leader of the team. "Subinvestigator" includes any other individual member of that team.

Marketing application means an application for a new drug submitted under section 505(b) of the Act, a request to provide for certification of an antibiotic submitted under section 507 of the Act, or a product license application for a biological product submitted under the Public Health Service Act.

Sponsor means a person who takes responsibility for and initiates a clinical investigation. The sponsor may be an individual or pharmaceutical company, governmental agency, academic institution, private organization, or other organization. The sponsor does not actually conduct the investigation unless the sponsor is a sponsor-investigator. A person other than an individual that uses one or more of its own employees to conduct an investigation that it has initiated is a sponsor, not a sponsor-investigator, and the employees are investigators.

Sponsor-Investigator means an individual who both initiates and conducts an investigation, and under whose immediate direction the investigational drug is administered or dispensed. The term does not include any person other than an individual. The requirements applicable to a sponsor-investigator under this part include both those applicable to an investigator and a sponsor.

Subject means a human who participates in an investigation, either as a recipient of the investigational new drug or as a control. A subject may be a healthy human or a patient with a disease.

Sec. 312.6 Labeling of an investigational new drug.

(a) The immediate package of an investigational new drug intended for human use shall bear a label with the statement "Caution: New Drug—Limited by Federal (or United States) law to investigational use."

(b) The label or labeling of an investigational new drug shall not bear any statement that is false or misleading in any particular and shall not represent that the investigational new drug is safe or effective for the purposes for which it is being investigated.

Sec. 312.7 Promotion and charging for investigational drugs.

(a) Promotion of an investigational new drug. A sponsor or investigator, or any person acting on behalf of a sponsor or investigator, shall not represent in a promotional context that an investigational new drug is safe or effective for the purposes for which it is under investigation or otherwise promote the drug. This provision is not intended to restrict the full exchange of scientific information concerning the drug, including dissemination of scientific findings in scientific or lay media. Rather, its intent is to restrict promotional claims of safety or effectiveness of the drug for a use for which it is under investigation and to preclude commercialization of the drug before it is approved for commercial distribution.

(b) Commercial distribution of an investigational new drug. A sponsor or investigator shall not commercially distribute or test market an investigational new drug.

(c) Prolonging an investigation. A sponsor shall not unduly prolong an investigation after finding that the results of the investigation appear to establish sufficient data to support a marketing application.

(d) Charging for and commercialization of investigational drugs—(1) Clinical trials under an IND. Charging for an investigational drug in a clinical trial under an IND is not permitted without the prior written approval of FDA. In requesting such approval, the sponsor shall provide a full written explanation of why charging is necessary in order for the sponsor to undertake or continue the clinical trial, e.g., why distribution of the drug to test subjects should not be considered part of the normal cost of doing business.

(2) Treatment protocol or treatment IND. A sponsor or investigator may charge for an investigational drug for a treatment use under a treatment protocol or treatment IND provided: (i) There is adequate enrollment in the ongoing clinical investigations under the authorized IND; (ii) charging does not constitute commercial marketing of a new drug for which a marketing application has not been approved; (iii) the drug is not being commercially promoted or advertised; and (iv) the sponsor of the drug is actively pursuing marketing approval with due diligence. FDA must be notified in writing in advance of commencing any such charges, in an information amendment submitted under Sec. 312.31. Authorization for charging goes into effect automatically 30 days after receipt by FDA of the information amendment, unless the sponsor is notified to the contrary.

(3) Noncommercialization of investigational drug. Under this section, the sponsor may not commercialize an investigational drug by charging a price larger than that necessary to recover costs of manufacture, research, development, and handling of the investigational drug.

(4) Withdrawal of authorization. Authorization to charge for an investigational drug under this section may be withdrawn by FDA if the agency finds that the conditions underlying the authorization are no longer satisfied.

(Collection of information requirements approved by the Office of Management and Budget under control number 0910-0014)

[52 FR 8831, Mar. 19, 1987, as amended at 52 FR 19476, May 22, 1987]

Sec. 312.10 Waivers.

(a) A sponsor may request FDA to waive applicable requirement under this part. A waiver request may be submitted either in an IND or in an information amendment to an IND. In an emergency, a request may be made by telephone or other rapid communication means. A waiver request is required to contain at least one of the following:

(1) An explanation why the sponsor's compliance with the requirement is unnecessary or cannot be achieved;

(2) A description of an alternative submission or course of action that satisfies the purpose of the requirement; or

(3) Other information justifying a waiver.

(b) FDA may grant a waiver if it finds that the sponsor's noncompliance would not pose a significant and unreasonable risk to human subjects of the investigation and that one of the following is met:

(1) The sponsor's compliance with the requirement is unnecessary for the agency to evaluate the application, or compliance cannot be achieved;

(2) The sponsor's proposed alternative satisfies the requirement; or

(3) The applicant's submission otherwise justifies a waiver.

(Collection of information requirements approved by the Office of Management and Budget under control number 0910-0014)

[52 FR 8831, Mar. 19, 1987, as amended at 52 FR 23031, June 17, 1987]

Subpart B—Investigational New Drug Application (IND)

Sec. 312.20 Requirement for an IND.

(a) A sponsor shall submit an IND to FDA if the sponsor intends to conduct a clinical investigation with an investigational new drug that is subject to Sec. 312.2(a).

(b) A sponsor shall not begin a clinical investigation subject to Sec. 312.2(a) until the investigation is subject to an IND which is in effect in accordance with Sec. 312.40.

(c) A sponsor shall submit a separate IND for any clinical investigation involving an exception from informed consent under Sec. 50.24 of this chapter. Such a clinical investigation is not permitted to proceed without the prior written authorization from FDA.

FDA shall provide a written determination 30 days after FDA receives the IND or earlier.

[52 FR 8831, Mar. 19, 1987, as amended at 61 FR 51529, Oct. 2, 1996; 62 FR 32479, June 16, 1997]

Sec. 312.21 Phases of an investigation.

An IND may be submitted for one or more phases of an investigation. The clinical investigation of a previously untested drug is generally divided into three phases. Although in general the phases are conducted sequentially, they may overlap. These three phases of an investigation are a follows:

(a) Phase 1. (1) Phase 1 includes the initial introduction of an investigational new drug into humans. Phase 1 studies are typically closely monitored and may be conducted in patients or normal volunteer subjects. These studies are designed to determine the metabolism and pharmacologic actions of the drug in humans, the side effects associated with increasing doses, and, if possible, to gain early evidence on effectiveness. During Phase 1, sufficient information about the drug's pharmacokinetics and pharmacological effects should be obtained to permit the design of well-controlled, scientifically valid, Phase 2 studies. The total number of subjects and patients included in Phase 1 studies varies with the drug, but is generally in the range of 20 to 80.

(2) Phase 1 studies also include studies of drug metabolism, structure-activity relationships, and mechanism of action in humans, as well as studies in which investigational drugs are used as research tools to explore biological phenomena or disease processes.

(b) Phase 2. Phase 2 includes the controlled clinical studies conducted to evaluate the effectiveness of the drug for a particular indication or indications in patients with the disease or condition under study and to determine the common short-term side effects and risks associated with the drug. Phase 2 studies are typically well controlled, closely monitored, and conducted in a relatively small number of patients, usually involving no more than several hundred subjects.

(c) Phase 3. Phase 3 studies are expanded controlled and uncontrolled trials. They are performed after preliminary evidence suggesting effectiveness of the drug has been obtained, and are intended to gather the additional information about effectiveness and safety that is needed to evaluate the overall benefit-risk relationship of the drug and to provide an adequate basis for physician labeling. Phase 3 studies usually include from several hundred to several thousand subjects.

Sec. 312.22 General principles of the IND submission.

(a) FDA's primary objectives in reviewing an IND are, in all phases of the investigation, to assure the safety and rights of subjects, and, in Phase 2 and 3, to help assure that the quality of the scientific evaluation of drugs is adequate to permit an evaluation of the drug's effectiveness and safety. Therefore, although FDA's review of Phase 1 submissions will focus on assessing the safety of Phase 1 investigations, FDA's review of Phases 2 and 3 submissions will also include an assessment of the scientific quality of the clinical investigations and the likelihood that the investigations will yield data capable of meeting statutory standards for marketing approval.

(b) The amount of information on a particular drug that must be submitted in an IND to assure the accomplishment of the objectives described in paragraph (a) of this section depends upon such factors as the novelty of the drug, the extent to which it has been studied previously, the known or suspected risks, and the developmental phase of the drug.

(c) The central focus of the initial IND submission should be on the general investigational plan and the protocols for specific human studies. Subsequent amendments to the IND that contain new or revised protocols should build logically on previous submissions and should be supported by additional information, including the results of animal toxicology studies or other human studies as appropriate. Annual reports to the IND should serve as the focus for reporting the status of studies being conducted under the IND and should update the general investigational plan for the coming year.

(d) The IND format set forth in Sec. 312.23 should be followed routinely by sponsors in the interest of fostering an efficient review of applications. Sponsors are expected to exercise considerable discretion, however, regarding the content of information submitted in each section, depending upon the kind of drug being studied and the nature of the available information. Section 312.23 outlines the information needed for a commercially sponsored IND for a new molecular entity. A sponsor-investigator who uses, as a research tool, an investigational new drug that is already subject to a manufacturer's IND or marketing application should follow the same general format, but ordinarily may, if authorized by the manufacturer, refer to the manufacturer's IND or marketing application in providing the technical information supporting the proposed clinical investigation. A sponsor-investigator who uses an investigational drug not subject to a manufacturer's IND or marketing application is ordinarily required to submit all technical information supporting the IND, unless such information may be referenced from the scientific literature.

Sec. 312.23 IND content and format.

(a) A sponsor who intends to conduct a clinical investigation subject to this part shall submit an "Investigational New Drug Application" (IND) including, in the following order:

(1) Cover sheet (Form FDA-1571). A cover sheet for the application containing the following:

(i) The name, address, and telephone number of the sponsor, the date of the application, and the name of the investigational new drug.

(ii) Identification of the phase or phases of the clinical investigation to be conducted.

(iii) A commitment not to begin clinical investigations until an IND covering the investigations is in effect.

(iv) A commitment that an Institutional Review Board (IRB) that complies with the requirements set forth in part 56 will be responsible for the initial and continuing review and approval of each of the studies in the proposed clinical investigation and that the investigator will report to the IRB proposed changes in the research activity in accordance with the requirements of part 56.

(v) A commitment to conduct the investigation in accordance with all other applicable regulatory requirements.

(vi) The name and title of the person responsible for monitoring the conduct and progress of the clinical investigations.

(vii) The name(s) and title(s) of the person(s) responsible under Sec. 312.32 for review and evaluation of information relevant to the safety of the drug.

(viii) If a sponsor has transferred any obligations for the conduct of any clinical study to a contract research organization, a statement containing the name and address of the contract research organization, identification of the clinical study, and a listing of the obligations transferred. If all obligations governing the conduct of the study have been transferred, a general statement of this transfer—in lieu of a listing of the specific obligations transferred—may be submitted.

(ix) The signature of the sponsor or the sponsor's authorized representative. If the person signing the application does not reside or have a place of business within the United States, the IND is required to contain the name and address of, and be countersigned by, an attorney, agent, or other authorized official who resides or maintains a place of business within the United States.

(2) A table of contents.

(3) Introductory statement and general investigational plan. (i) A brief introductory statement giving the name of the drug and all active ingredients, the drug's pharmacological class, the structural formula of the drug (if known), the formulation of the dosage form(s) to be used, the route of administration, and the broad objectives and planned duration of the proposed clinical investigation(s).

(ii) A brief summary of previous human experience with the drug, with reference to other IND's if pertinent, and to investigational or marketing experience in other countries that may be relevant to the safety of the proposed clinical investigation(s).

(iii) If the drug has been withdrawn from investigation or marketing in any country for any reason related to safety or effectiveness, identification of the country(ies) where the drug was withdrawn and the reasons for the withdrawal.

(iv) A brief description of the overall plan for investigating the drug product for the following year. The plan should include the following: (a) The rationale for the drug or the research study; (b) the indication(s) to be studied; (c) the general approach to be followed in evaluating the drug; (d) the kinds of clinical trials to be conducted in the first year following the submission (if plans are not developed for the entire year, the sponsor should so indicate); (e) the estimated number of patients to be given the drug in those studies; and (f) any risks of particular severity or seriousness anticipated on the basis of the toxicological data in animals or prior studies in humans with the drug or related drugs.

(4) [Reserved]

(5) Investigator's brochure. If required under Sec. 312.55, a copy of the investigator's brochure, containing the following information:

(i) A brief description of the drug substance and the formulation, including the structural formula, if known.

(ii) A summary of the pharmacological and toxicological effects of the drug in animals and, to the extent known, in humans.

(iii) A summary of the pharmacokinetics and biological disposition of the drug in animals and, if known, in humans.

(iv) A summary of information relating to safety and effectiveness in humans obtained from prior clinical studies. (Reprints of published articles on such studies may be appended when useful.)

(v) A description of possible risks and side effects to be anticipated on the basis of prior experience with the drug under investigation or with related drugs, and of precautions or special monitoring to be done as part of the investigational use of the drug.

(6) Protocols. (i) A protocol for each planned study. (Protocols for studies not submitted initially in the IND should be submitted in accordance with Sec. 312.30(a).) In general, protocols for Phase 1 studies may be less detailed and more flexible than protocols for Phase 2 and 3 studies. Phase 1 protocols should be directed primarily at providing an outline of the investigation—an estimate of the number of patients to be involved, a description of safety exclusions, and a description of the dosing plan including duration, dose, or method to be used in determining dose—and should specify in detail only those elements of the study that are critical to safety, such as necessary monitoring of vital signs and blood chemistries. Modifications of the experimental design of Phase 1 studies that do not affect critical safety assessments are required to be reported to FDA only in the annual report.

(ii) In Phases 2 and 3, detailed protocols describing all aspects of the study should be submitted. A protocol for a Phase 2 or 3 investigation should be designed in such a way that, if the sponsor anticipates that some deviation from the study design may become necessary as the investigation progresses, alternatives or contingencies to provide for such deviation are built into the protocols at the outset. For example, a protocol for a controlled short-term study might include a plan for an early crossover of nonresponders to an alternative therapy.

(iii) A protocol is required to contain the following, with the specific elements and detail of the protocol reflecting the above distinctions depending on the phase of study:

(a) A statement of the objectives and purpose of the study.

(b) The name and address and a statement of the qualifications (curriculum vitae or other statement of qualifications) of each investigator, and the name of each subinvestigator (e.g., research fellow, resident) working under the supervision of the investigator; the name and address of the research facilities to be used; and the name and address of each reviewing Institutional Review Board.

(c) The criteria for patient selection and for exclusion of patients and an estimate of the number of patients to be studied.

(d) A description of the design of the study, including the kind of control group to be used, if any, and a description of methods to be used to minimize bias on the part of subjects, investigators, and analysts.

(e) The method for determining the dose(s) to be administered, the planned maximum dosage, and the duration of individual patient exposure to the drug.

(f) A description of the observations and measurements to be made to fulfill the objectives of the study.

(g) A description of clinical procedures, laboratory tests, or other measures to be taken to monitor the effects of the drug in human subjects and to minimize risk.

(7) Chemistry, manufacturing, and control information. (i) As appropriate for the particular investigations covered by the IND, a section describing the composition, manufacture, and control of the drug substance and the drug product. Although in each phase of the investigation sufficient information is required to be submitted to assure the proper identification, quality, purity, and strength of the investigational drug, the amount of information needed to make that assurance will vary with the phase of the investigation, the proposed duration of the investigation, the dosage form, and the amount of information otherwise available. FDA recognizes that modifications to the method of preparation of the new drug substance and dosage form and changes in the dosage form itself are likely as the investigation progresses. Therefore, the emphasis in an initial Phase 1 submission should generally be placed on the identification and control of the raw materials and the new drug substance. Final specifications for the drug substance and drug product are not expected until the end of the investigational process.

(ii) It should be emphasized that the amount of information to be submitted depends upon the scope of the proposed clinical investigation. For example, although stability data are required in all phases of the IND to demonstrate that the new drug substance and drug product are within acceptable chemical and physical limits for the planned duration of the proposed clinical investigation, if very short-term tests are proposed, the supporting stability data can be correspondingly limited.

(iii) As drug development proceeds and as the scale or production is changed from the pilot-scale production appropriate for the limited initial clinical investigations to the larger-scale production needed for expanded clinical trials, the sponsor should submit information amendments to supplement the initial information submitted on the chemistry, manufacturing, and control processes with information appropriate to the expanded scope of the investigation.

(iv) Reflecting the distinctions described in this paragraph (a)(7), and based on the phase(s) to be studied, the submission is required to contain the following:

(a) Drug substance. A description of the drug substance, including its physical, chemical, or biological characteristics; the name and address of its manufacturer; the general method of preparation of the drug substance; the acceptable limits and analytical methods used to assure the identity, strength, quality, and purity of the drug substance; and information sufficient to support stability of the drug substance during the toxicological studies and the planned clinical studies. Reference to the current edition of the United States Pharmacopeia—National Formulary may satisfy relevant requirements in this paragraph.

(b) Drug product. A list of all components, which may include reasonable alternatives for inactive compounds, used in the manufacture of the investigational drug product, including both those components intended to appear in the drug product and those which may not appear but which are used in the manufacturing process, and, where applicable, the quantitative composition of the investigational drug product, including any reasonable variations that may be expected during the investigational stage; the name and address of the drug product manufacturer; a brief general description of the manufacturing and packaging procedure as appropriate for the product; the acceptable limits and analytical methods used to assure the identity, strength, quality, and purity of the drug product; and information sufficient to assure the product's stability during the planned clinical studies. Reference to the current edition of the United States Pharmacopeia—National Formulary may satisfy certain requirements in this paragraph.

(c) A brief general description of the composition, manufacture, and control of any placebo used in a controlled clinical trial.

(d) Labeling. A copy of all labels and labeling to be provided to each investigator.

(e) Environmental analysis requirements. A claim for categorical exclusion under Sec. 25.30 or 25.31 or an environmental assessment under Sec. 25.40.

(8) Pharmacology and toxicology information. Adequate information about pharmacological and toxicological studies of the drug involving laboratory animals or in vitro, on the basis of which the sponsor has concluded that it is reasonably safe to conduct the proposed clinical investigations. The kind, duration, and scope of animal and other tests required varies with the duration and nature of the proposed clinical investigations. Guidelines are available from FDA that describe ways in which these requirements may be met. Such information is required to include the identification and qualifications of the individuals who evaluated the results of such studies and concluded that it is reasonably safe to begin the proposed investigations and a statement of where the investigations were conducted and where the records are available for inspection. As drug development proceeds, the sponsor is required to submit informational amendments, as appropriate, with additional information pertinent to safety.

(i) Pharmacology and drug disposition. A section describing the pharmacological effects and mechanism(s) of action of the drug in animals, and information on the absorption, distribution, metabolism, and excretion of the drug, if known.

(ii) Toxicology. (a) An integrated summary of the toxicological effects of the drug in animals and in vitro. Depending on the nature of the drug and the phase of the investigation, the description is to include the results of acute, subacute, and chronic toxicity tests; tests of the drug's effects on reproduction and the developing fetus; any special toxicity test related to the drug's particular mode of administration or conditions of use (e.g., inhalation, dermal, or ocular toxicology); and any in vitro studies intended to evaluate drug toxicity.

(b) For each toxicology study that is intended primarily to support the safety of the proposed clinical investigation, a full tabulation of data suitable for detailed review.

(iii) For each nonclinical laboratory study subject to the good laboratory practice regulations under part 58, a statement that the study was conducted in compliance with the good laboratory practice regulations in part 58, or, if the study was not conducted in compliance with those regulations, a brief statement of the reason for the noncompliance.

(9) Previous human experience with the investigational drug. A summary of previous human experience known to the applicant, if any, with the investigational drug. The information is required to include the following:

(i) If the investigational drug has been investigated or marketed previously, either in the United States or other countries, detailed information about such experience that is relevant to the safety of the proposed investigation or to the investigation's rationale. If the durg has been the subject of controlled trials, detailed information on such trials that is relevant to an assessment of the drug's effectiveness for the proposed investigational use(s) should also be provided. Any published material that is relevant to the safety of the proposed investigation or to an assessment of the drug's effectiveness for its proposed investigational use should be provided in full. Published material that is less directly relevant may be supplied by a bibliography.

(ii) If the drug is a combination of drugs previously investigated or marketed, the information required under paragraph (a)(9)(i) of this section should be provided for each active drug component. However, if any component in such combination is subject to an approved marketing application or is otherwise lawfully marketed in the United States, the sponsor is not required to submit published material concerning that active drug component unless such material relates directly to the proosed investigational use (including publications relevant to component-component interaction).

(iii) If the drug has been marketed outside the United States, a list of the countries in which the drug has been marketed and a list of the countries in which the drug has been withdrawn from marketing for reasons potentially related to safety or effectiveness.

(10) Additional information. In certain applications, as described below, information on special topics may be needed. Such information shall be submitted in this section as follows:

(i) Drug dependence and abuse potential. If the drug is a psychotropic substance or otherwise has abuse potential, a section describing relevant clinical studies and experience and studies in test animals.

(ii) Radioactive drugs. If the drug is a radioactive drug, sufficient data from animal or human studies to allow a reasonable calculation of radiation-absorbed dose to the whole body and critical organs upon administration to a human subject. Phase 1 studies of radioactive drugs must include studies which will obtain sufficient data for dosimetry calculations.

(iii) Other information. A brief statement of any other information that would aid evaluation of the proposed clinical investigations with respect to their safety or their design and potential as controlled clinical trials to support marketing of the drug.

(11) Relevant information. If requested by FDA, any other relevant information needed for review of the application.

(b) Information previously submitted. The sponsor ordinarily is not required to resubmit information previously submitted, but may incorporate the information by reference. A reference to information submitted previously must identify the file by name, reference number, volume, and page number where the information can be found. A reference to information submitted to the agency by a person other than the sponsor is required to contain a written statement that authorizes he reference and that is signed by the person who submitted the information.

(c) Material in a foreign language. The sponsor shall submit an accurate and complete English translation of each part of the IND that is not in English. The sponsor shall also submit a copy of each original literature publication for which an English translation is submitted.

(d) Number of copies. The sponsor shall submit an original and two copies of all submissions to the IND file, including the original submission and all amendments and reports.

(e) Numbering of IND submissions. Each submission relating to an IND is required to be numbered serially using a single, three-digit serial number. The initial IND is required to be numbered 000; each subsequent submission (e.g., amendment, report, or correspondence) is required to be numbered chronologically in sequence.

(f) Identification of exception from informed consent. If the investigation involves an exception from informed consent under Sec. 50.24 of this chapter, the sponsor shall prominently identify on the cover sheet that the investigation is subject to the requirements in Sec. 50.24 of this chapter.

(Collection of information requirements approved by the Office of Management and Budget under control number 0910-0014)

[52 FR 8831, Mar. 19, 1987, as amended at 52 FR 23031, June 17, 1987; 53 FR 1918, Jan. 25, 1988; 61 FR 51529, Oct. 2, 1996; 62 FR 40599, July 29, 1997]

Sec. 312.30 Protocol amendments.

Once an IND is in effect, a sponsor shall amend it as needed to ensure that the clinical investigations are conducted according to protocols included in the application. This section sets forth the provisions under which new protocols may be submitted and changes in previously submitted protocols may be made. Whenever a sponsor intends to conduct a clinical investigation with an exception from informed consent for emergency research as set forth in Sec. 50.24 of this chapter, the sponsor shall submit a separate IND for such investigation.

(a) New protocol. Whenever a sponsor intends to conduct a study that is not covered by a protocol already contained in the IND, the sponsor shall submit to FDA a protocol amendment containing the protocol for the study. Such study may begin provided two conditions are met: (1) The sponsor has submitted the protocol to FDA for its review; and (2) the protocol has been approved by the Institutional Review Board (IRB) with responsibility for review and approval of the study in accordance with the requirements of part 56. The sponsor may comply with these two conditions in either order.

(b) Changes in a protocol. (1) A sponsor shall submit a protocol amendment describing any change in a Phase 1 protocol that significantly affects the safety of subjects or any change in a Phase 2 or 3 protocol that significantly affects the safety of subjects, the scope of the investigation, or the scientific quality of the study. Examples of changes requiring an amendment under this paragraph include:

(i) Any increase in drug dosage or duration of exposure of individual subjects to the drug beyond that in the current protocol, or any significant increase in the number of subjects under study.

(ii) Any significant change in the design of a protocol (such as the addition or dropping of a control group).

(iii) The addition of a new test or procedure that is intended to improve monitoring for, or reduce the risk of, a side effect or adverse event; or the dropping of a test intended to monitor safety.

(2)(i) A protocol change under paragraph (b)(1) of this section may be made provided two conditions are met:

(a) The sponsor has submitted the change to FDA for its review; and

(b) The change has been approved by the IRB with responsibility for review and approval of the study. The sponsor may comply with these two conditions in either order.

(ii) Notwithstanding paragraph (b)(2)(i) of this section, a protocol change intended to eliminate an apparent immediate hazard to subjects may be implemented immediately provided FDA is subsequently notified by protocol amendment and the reviewing IRB is notified in accordance with Sec. 56.104(c).

(c) New investigator. A sponsor shall submit a protocol amendment when a new investigator is added to carry out a previously submitted protocol, except that a protocol amendment is not required when a licensed practitioner is added in the case of a treatment protocol under Sec. 312.34. Once the investigator is added to the study, the investigational drug may be shipped to the investigator and the investigator may begin participating in the study.

The sponsor shall notify FDA of the new investigator within 30 days of the investigator being added.

(d) Content and format. A protocol amendment is required to be prominently identified as such (i.e., "Protocol Amendment: New Protocol", "Protocol Amendment: Change in Protocol", or "Protocol Amendment: New Investigator"), and to contain the following:

(1)(i) In the case of a new protocol, a copy of the new protocol and a brief description of the most clinically significant differences between it and previous protocols.

(ii) In the case of a change in protocol, a brief description of the change and reference (date and number) to the submission that contained the protocol.

(iii) In the case of a new investigator, the investigator's name, the qualifications to conduct the investigation, reference to the previously submitted protocol, and all additional information about the investigator's study as is required under Sec. 312.23(a)(6)(iii)(b).

(2) Reference, if necessary, to specific technical information in the IND or in a concurrently submitted information amendment to the IND that the sponsor relies on to support any clinically significant change in the new or amended protocol. If the reference is made to supporting information already in the IND, the sponsor shall identify by name, reference number, volume, and page number the location of the information.

(3) If the sponsor desires FDA to comment on the submission, a request for such comment and the specific questions FDA's response should address.

(e) When submitted. A sponsor shall submit a protocol amendment for a new protocol or a change in protocol before its implementation. Protocol amendments to add a new investigator or to provide additional information about investigators may be grouped and submitted at 30-dayintervals. When several submissions of new protocols or protocol changes are anticipated during a short period, the sponsor is encouraged, to the extent feasible, to include these all in a single submission.

(Collection of information requirements approved by the Office of Management and Budget under control number 0910-0014)

[52 FR 8831, Mar. 19, 1987, as amended at 52 FR 23031, June 17, 1987; 53 FR 1918, Jan. 25, 1988; 61 FR 51530, Oct. 2, 1996]

Sec. 312.31 Information amendments.

(a) Requirement for information amendment. A sponsor shall report in an information amendment essential information on the IND that is not within the scope of a protocol amendment, IND safety reports, or annual report. Examples of information requiring an information amendment include:

(1) New toxicology, chemistry, or other technical information; or

(2) A report regarding the discontinuance of a clinical investigation.

(b) Content and format of an information amendment. An information amendment is required to bear prominent identification of its contents (e.g., "Information Amendment: Chemistry, Manufacturing, and Control", "Information Amendment: Pharmacology-Toxicology", "Information Amendment: Clinical"), and to contain the following:

(1) A statement of the nature and purpose of the amendment.

(2) An organized submission of the data in a format appropriate for scientific review.

(3) If the sponsor desires FDA to comment on an information amendment, a request for such comment.

(c) When submitted. Information amendments to the IND should be submitted as necessary but, to the extent feasible, not more than every 30 days.

(Collection of information requirements approved by the Office of Management and Budget under control number 0910-0014)

[52 FR 8831, Mar. 19, 1987, as amended at 52 FR 23031, June 17, 1987; 53 FR 1918, Jan. 25, 1988]

Sec. 312.32 IND safety reports.

(a) Definitions. The following definitions of terms apply to this section: Associated with the use of the drug. There is a reasonable possibility that the experience may have been caused by the drug.

Disability. A substantial disruption of a person's ability to conduct normal life functions.

Life-threatening adverse drug experience. Any adverse drug experience that places the patient or subject, in the view of the investigator, at immediate risk of death from the reaction as it occurred, i.e., it does not include a reaction that, had it occurred in a more severe form, might have caused death.

Serious adverse drug experience: Any adverse drug experience occurring at any dose that results in any of the following outcomes: Death, a life-threatening adverse drug experience, inpatient hospitalization or prolongation of existing hospitalization, a persistent or significant disability/incapacity, or a congenital anomaly/birth defect. Important medical events that may not result in death, be life-threatening, or require hospitalization may be considered a serious adverse drug experience when, based upon appropriate medical judgment, they may jeopardize the patient or subject and may require medical or surgical intervention to prevent one of the outcomes listed in this definition. Examples of such medical events include allergic bronchospasm requiring intensive treatment in an emergency room or at home, blood dyscrasias or convulsions that do not result in inpatient hospitalization, or the development of drug dependency or drug abuse.

Unexpected adverse drug experience: Any adverse drug experience, the specificity or severity of which is not consistent with the current investigator brochure; or, if an investigator brochure is not required or available, the specificity or severity of which is not consistent with the risk information described in the general investigational plan or elsewhere in the current application, as amended. For example, under this definition, hepatic necrosis would be unexpected (by virtue of greater severity) if the investigator brochure only referred to elevated hepatic enzymes or hepatitis. Similarly, cerebral thromboembolism and cerebral vasculitis would be unexpected (by virtue of greater specificity) if the investigator brochure only listed cerebral vascular accidents. "Unexpected," as used in this definition, refers to an adverse drug experience that has not been previously observed (e.g., included in the investigator brochure) rather than from the perspective of such experience not being anticipated from the pharmacological properties of the pharmaceutical product.

(b) Review of safety information. The sponsor shall promptly review all information relevant to the safety of the drug obtained or otherwise received by the sponsor from any source, foreign or domestic, including information derived from any clinical or epidemiological investigations, animal investigations, commercial marketing experience, reports in the scientific literature, and unpublished scientific papers, as well as reports from foreign regulatory authorities that have not already been previously reported to the agency by the sponsor.

(c) IND safety reports. (1) Written reports—(i) The sponsor shall notify FDA and all participating investigators in a written IND safety report of:

(A) Any adverse experience associated with the use of the drug that is both serious and unexpected; or

(B) Any finding from tests in laboratory animals that suggests a significant risk for human subjects including reports of mutagenicity, teratogenicity, or carcinogenicity. Each notification shall be made as soon as possible and in no event later than 15 calendar days after the sponsor's initial receipt of the information. Each written notification may be submitted on FDA Form 3500A or in a narrative format (foreign events may be submitted either on an FDA Form 3500A or, if preferred, on a CIOMS I form; reports from animal or epidemiological studies shall be submitted in a narrative format) and shall bear prominent identification of its contents, i.e., "IND Safety Report." Each written notification to FDA shall be transmitted to the FDA new drug review division in the Center for Drug Evaluation and Research or the product review division in the Center for Biologics Evaluation and Research that has responsibility for review of the IND. If FDA determines that additional data are needed, the agency may require further data to be submitted.

(ii) In each written IND safety report, the sponsor shall identify all safety reports previously filed with the IND concerning a similar adverse experience, and shall analyze the significance of the adverse experience in light of the previous, similar reports.

(2) Telephone and facsimile transmission safety reports. The sponsor shall also notify FDA by telephone or by facsimile transmission of any unexpected fatal or life-threatening experience associated with the use of the drug as soon as possible but in no event later than 7 calendar days after the sponsor's initial receipt of the information. Each telephone call or facsimile transmission to FDA shall be transmitted to the FDA new drug review division in the Center for Drug Evaluation and Research or the product review division in the Center for Biologics Evaluation and Research that has responsibility for review of the IND.

(3) Reporting format or frequency. FDA may request a sponsor to submit IND safety reports in a format or at a frequency different than that required under this paragraph. The sponsor may also propose and adopt a different reporting format or frequency if the change is agreed to in advance by the director of the new drug review division in the Center for Drug Evaluation and Research or the director of the products review division in the Center for Biologics Evaluation and Research which is responsible for review of the IND.

(4) A sponsor of a clinical study of a marketed drug is not required to make a safety report for any adverse experience associated with use of the drug that is not from the clinical study itself.

(d) Followup. (1) The sponsor shall promptly investigate all safety information received by it.

(2) Followup information to a safety report shall be submitted as soon as the relevant information is available.

(3) If the results of a sponsor's investigation show that an adverse drug experience not initially determined to be reportable under paragraph (c) of this section is so reportable, the sponsor shall report such experience in a written safety report as soon as possible, but in no event later than 15 calendar days after the determination is made.

(4) Results of a sponsor's investigation of other safety information shall be submitted, as appropriate, in an information amendment or annual report.

(e) Disclaimer. A safety report or other information submitted by a sponsor under this part (and any release by FDA of that report or information) does not necessarily reflect a conclusion by the sponsor or FDA that the report or information constitutes an admission that the drug caused or contributed to an adverse experience. A sponsor need not admit, and may deny, that the report or information submitted by the sponsor constitutes an admission that the drug caused or contributed to an adverse experience.

(Collection of information requirements approved by the Office of Management and Budget under control number 0910-0014)

[52 FR 8831, Mar. 19, 1987, as amended at 52 FR 23031, June 17, 1987; 55 FR 11579, Mar. 29, 1990; 62 FR 52250, Oct. 7, 1997]

Effective Date Note: At 62 FR 52250, Oct. 7, 1997, Sec. 312.32 was amended by revising paragraphs (a), (b), (c)(1)(i), (c)(2), and (d)(3); by adding in the second sentence of paragraph (c)(3) the words "new drug review" before the phrase "division in the Center for Drug Evaluation and Research" and the words "the director of the product review division in" before the phrase "the Center for Biologics Evaluation and Research"; and by removing in paragraph (e) the word "section" and replacing it with the word "part", effective Apr. 6, 1998.

Sec. 312.33 Annual reports.

A sponsor shall within 60 days of the anniversary date that the IND went into effect, submit a brief report of the progress of the investigation that includes:

(a) Individual study information. A brief summary of the status of each study in progress and each study completed during the previous year. The summary is required to include the following information for each study:

(1) The title of the study (with any appropriate study identifiers such as protocol num-

ber), its purpose, a brief statement identifying the patient population, and a statement as to whether the study is completed.

(2) The total number of subjects initially planned for inclusion in the study; the number entered into the study to date, tabulated by age group, gender, and race; the number whose participation in the study was completed as planned; and the number who dropped out of the study for any reason.

(3) If the study has been completed, or if interim results are known, a brief description of any available study results.

(b) Summary information. Information obtained during the previous year's clinical and nonclinical investigations, including:

(1) A narrative or tabular summary showing the most frequent and most serious adverse experiences by body system.

(2) A summary of all IND safety reports submitted during the past year.

(3) A list of subjects who died during participation in the investigation, with the cause of death for each subject.

(4) A list of subjects who dropped out during the course of the investigation in association with any adverse experience, whether or not thought to be drug related.

(5) A brief description of what, if anything, was obtained that is pertinent to an understanding of the drug's actions, including, for example, information about dose response, information from controlled trails, and information about bioavailability.

(6) A list of the preclinical studies (including animal studies) completed or in progress during the past year and a summary of the major preclinical findings.

(7) A summary of any significant manufacturing or microbiological changes made during the past year.

(c) A description of the general investigational plan for the coming year to replace that submitted 1 year earlier. The general investigational plan shall contain the information required under Sec. 312.23(a)(3)(iv).

(d) If the investigator brochure has been revised, a description of the revision and a copy of the new brochure.

(e) A description of any significant Phase 1 protocol modifications made during the previous year and not previously reported to the IND ina protocol amendment.

(f) A brief summary of significant foreign marketing developments with the drug during the past year, such as approval of marketing in any country or withdrawal or suspension from marketing in any country.

(g) If desired by the sponsor, a log of any outstanding business with respect to the IND for which the sponsor requests or expects a reply, comment, or meeting.

(Collection of information requirements approved by the Office of Management and Budget under control number 0910-0014)

[52 FR 8831, Mar. 19, 1987, as amended at 52 FR 23031, June 17, 1987; 63 FR 6862, Feb. 11, 1998]

Effective Date Note: At 63 FR 6862, Feb. 11, 1998, Sec. 312.33 was amended by revising paragraph (a)(2), effective Aug. 10, 1998.

Sec. 312.34 Treatment use of an investigational new drug.

(a) General. A drug that is not approved for marketing may be under clinical investigation for a serious or immediately life-threatening disease condition in patients for whom no comparable or satisfactory alternative drug or other therapy is available. During the clinical investigation of the drug, it may be appropriate to use the drug in the treatment of patients not in the clinical trials, in accordance with a treatment protocol or treatment IND. The purpose of this section is to facilitate the availability of promising new drugs to desperately ill patients as early in the drug development process as possible, before general marketing begins, and to obtain additional data on the drug's safety and effectiveness. In the case of a serious disease, a drug ordinarily may be made available for treatment use under this section during

Phase 3 investigations or after all clinical trials have been completed; however, in appropriate circumstances, a drug may be made available for treatment use during Phase 2. In the case of an immediately life-threatening disease, a drug may be made available for treatment use under this section earlier than Phase 3, but ordinarily not earlier than Phase 2. For purposes of this section, the "treatment use" of a drug includes the use of a drug for diagnostic purposes. If a protocol for an investigational drug meets the criteria of this section, the protocol is to be submitted as a treatment protocol under the provisions of this section.

(b) Criteria. (1) FDA shall permit an investigational drug to be used for a treatment use under a treatment protocol or treatment IND if:

(i) The drug is intended to treat a serious or immediately life-threatening disease;

(ii) There is no comparable or satisfactory alternative drug or other therapy available to treat that stage of the disease in the intended patient population;

(iii) The drug is under investigation in a controlled clinical trial under an IND in effect for the trial, or all clinical trials have been completed; and

(iv) The sponsor of the controlled clinical trial is actively pursuing marketing approval of the investigational drug with due diligence.

(2) Serious disease. For a drug intended to treat a serious disease, the Commissioner may deny a request for treatment use under a treatment protocol or treatment IND if there is insufficient evidence of safety and effectiveness to support such use.

(3) Immediately life-threatening disease. (i) For a drug intended to treat an immediately life-threatening disease, the Commissioner may deny a request for treatment use of an investigational drug under a treatment protocol or treatment IND if the available scientific evidence, taken as a whole, fails to provide a reasonable basis for concluding that the drug:

(A) May be effective for its intended use in its intended patient population; or

(B) Would not expose the patients to whom the drug is to be administered to an unreasonable and significant additional risk of illness or injury.

(ii) For the purpose of this section, an "immediately life-threatening" disease means a stage of a disease in which there is a reasonable likelihood that death will occur within a matter of months or in which premature death is likely without early treatment.

(c) Safeguards. Treatment use of an investigational drug is conditioned on the sponsor and investigators complying with the safeguards of the IND process, including the regulations governing informed consent (21 CFR part 50) and institutional review boards (21 CFR part 56) and the applicable provisions of part 312, including distribution of the drug through qualified experts, maintenance of adequate manufacturing facilities, and submission of IND safety reports.

(d) Clinical hold. FDA may place on clinical hold a proposed or ongoing treatment protocol or treatment IND in accordance with Sec. 312.42.

[52 FR 19476, May 22, 1987, as amended at 57 FR 13248, Apr. 15, 1992]

Sec. 312.35 Submissions for treatment use.

(a) Treatment protocol submitted by IND sponsor. Any sponsor of a clinical investigation of a drug who intends to sponsor a treatment use for the drug shall submit to FDA a treatment protocol under Sec. 312.34 if the sponsor believes the criteria of Sec. 312.34 are satisfied. If a protocol is not submitted under Sec. 312.34, but FDA believes that the protocol should have been submitted under this section, FDA may deem the protocol to be submitted under Sec. 312.34. A treatment use under a treatment protocol may begin 30 days after FDA receives the protocol or on earlier notification by FDA that the treatment use described in the protocol may begin.

(1) A treatment protocol is required to contain the following:

(i) The intended use of the drug.

(ii) An explanation of the rationale for use of the drug, including, as appropriate, either a list of what available regimens ordinarily should be tried before using the investigational drug or an explanation of why the use of the investigational drug is preferable to the use of available marketed treatments.

(iii) A brief description of the criteria for patient selection.

(iv) The method of administration of the drug and the dosages.

(v) A description of clinical procedures, laboratory tests, or other measures to monitor the effects of the drug and to minimize risk.

(2) A treatment protocol is to be supported by the following:

(i) Informational brochure for supplying to each treating physician.

(ii) The technical information that is relevant to safety and effectiveness of the drug for the intended treatment purpose. Information contained in the sponsor's IND may be incorporated by reference.

(iii) A commitment by the sponsor to assure compliance of all participating investigators with the informed consent requirements of 21 CFR part 50.

(3) A licensed practiner who receives an investigational drug for treatment use under a treatment protocol is an "investigator" under the protocol and is responsible for meeting all applicable investigator responsibilities under this part and 21 CFR parts 50 and 56.

(b) Treatment IND submitted by licensed practitioner. (1) If a licensed medical practitioner wants to obtain an investigational drug subject to a controlled clinical trial for a treatment use, the practitioner should first attempt to obtain the drug from the sponsor of the controlled trial under a treatment protocol. If the sponsor of the controlled clinical investigation of the drug will not establish a treatment protocol for the drug under paragraph (a) of this section, the licensed medical practitioner may seek to obtain the drug from the sponsor and submit a treatment IND to FDA requesting authorization to use the investigational drug for treatment use. A treatment use under a treatment IND may begin 30 days after FDA receives the IND or on earlier notification by FDA that the treatment use under the IND may begin. A treatment IND is required to contain the following:

(i) A cover sheet (Form FDA 1571) meeting Sec. 312.23(g)(1).

(ii) Information (when not provided by the sponsor) on the drug's chemistry, manufacturing, and controls, and prior clinical and nonclinical experience with the drug submitted in accordance with Sec. 312.23. A sponsor of a clinical investigation subject to an IND who supplies an investigational drug to a licensed medical practitioner for purposes of a separate treatment clinical investigation shall be deemed to authorize the incorporation-by-reference of the technical information contained in the sponsor's IND into the medical practitioner's treatment IND.

(iii) A statement of the steps taken by the practitioner to obtain the drug under a treatment protocol from the drug sponsor.

(iv) A treatment protocol containing the same information listed in paragraph (a)(1) of this section.

(v) A statement of the practitioner's qualifications to use the investigational drug for the intended treatment use.

(vi) The practitioner's statement of familiarity with information on the drug's safety and effectiveness derived from previous clinical and nonclinical experience with the drug.

(vii) Agreement to report to FDA safety information in accordance with Sec. 312.32.

(2) A licensed practitioner who submits a treatment IND under this section is the sponsor-investigator for such IND and is responsible for meeting all applicable sponsor and investigator responsibilities under this part and 21 CFR parts 50 and 56.

(Collection of information requirements approved by the Office of Management and Budget under control number 0910-0014)

[52 FR 19477, May 22, 1987, as amended at 57 FR 13249, Apr. 15, 1992]

Sec. 312.36 Emergency use of an investigational new drug.

Need for an investigational drug may arise in an emergency situation that does not allow time for submission of an IND in accordance with Sec. 312.23 or Sec. 312.34. In such a case, FDA may authorize shipment of the drug for a specified use in advance of submission of an IND. A request for such authorization may be transmitted to FDA by telephone or other rapid communication means. For investigational biological drugs, the request should be directed to the Division of Biological Investigational New Drugs (HFB-230), Center for Biologics Evaluation and Research, 8800 Rockville Pike, Bethesda, MD 20892, 301-443-4864. For all other investigational drugs, the request for authorization should be directed to the Document Management and Reporting Branch (HFD-53), Center for Drug Evaluation and Research, 5600 Fishers Lane, Rockville, MD 20857, 301-443-4320. After normal working hours, eastern standard time, the request should be directed to the FDA Division of Emergency and Epidemiological Operations, 202-857-8400. Except in extraordinary circumstances, such authorization will be conditioned on the sponsor making an appropriate IND submission as soon as practicable after receiving the authorization.

(Collection of information requirements approved by the Office of Management and Budget under control number 0910-0014)

[52 FR 8831, Mar. 19, 1987, as amended at 52 FR 23031, June 17, 1987; 55 FR 11579, Mar. 29, 1990]

Sec. 312.38 Withdrawal of an IND.

(a) At any time a sponsor may withdraw an effective IND without prejudice.

(b) If an IND is withdrawn, FDA shall be so notified, all clinical investigations conducted under the IND shall be ended, all current investigators notified, and all stocks of the drug returned to the sponsor or otherwise disposed of at the request of the sponsor in accordance with Sec. 312.59.

(c) If an IND is withdrawn because of a safety reason, the sponsor shall promptly so inform FDA, all participating investigators, and all reviewing Institutional Review Boards, together with the reasons for such withdrawal.

(Collection of information requirements approved by the Office of Management and Budget under control number 0910-0014)

[52 FR 8831, Mar. 19, 1987, as amended at 52 FR 23031, June 17, 1987]

Subpart C—Administrative Actions

Sec. 312.40 General requirements for use of an investigational new drug in a clinical investigation.

(a) An investigational new drug may be used in a clinical investigation if the following conditions are met:

(1) The sponsor of the investigation submits an IND for the drug to FDA; the IND is in effect under paragraph (b) of this section; and the sponsor complies with all applicable requirements in this part and parts 50 and 56 with respect to the conduct of the clinical investigations; and

(2) Each participating investigator conducts his or her investigation in compliance with the requirements of this part and parts 50 and 56.

(b) An IND goes into effect:

(1) Thirty days after FDA receives the IND, unless FDA notifies the sponsor that the investigations described in the IND are subject to a clinical hold under Sec. 312.42; or

(2) On earlier notification by FDA that the clinical investigations in the IND may begin. FDA will notify the sponsor in writing of the date it receives the IND.

(c) A sponsor may ship an investigational new drug to investigators named in the IND:

(1) Thirty days after FDA receives the IND; or

(2) On earlier FDA authorization to ship the drug.

(d) An investigator may not administer an investigational new drug to human subjects until the IND goes into effect under paragraph (b) of this section.

Sec. 312.41 Comment and advice on an IND.

(a) FDA may at any time during the course of the investigation communicate with the sponsor orally or in writing about deficiencies in the IND or about FDA's need for more data or information.

(b) On the sponsor's request, FDA will provide advice on specific matters relating to an IND. Examples of such advice may include advice on the adequacy of technical data to support an investigational plan, on the design of a clinical trial, and on whether proposed investigations are likely to produce the data and information that is needed to meet requirements for a marketing application.

(c) Unless the communication is accompanied by a clinical hold order under Sec. 312.42, FDA communications with a sponsor under this section are solely advisory and do not require any modification in the planned or ongoing clinical investigations or response to the agency.

(Collection of information requirements approved by the Office of Management and Budget under control number 0910-0014)

[52 FR 8831, Mar. 19, 1987, as amended at 52 FR 23031, June 17, 1987]

Sec. 312.42 Clinical holds and requests for modification.

(a) General. A clinical hold is an order issued by FDA to the sponsor to delay a proposed clinical investigation or to suspend an ongoing investigation. The clinical hold order may apply to one or more of the investigations covered by an IND. When a proposed study is placed on clinical hold, subjects may not be given the investigational drug. When an ongoing study is placed on clinical hold, no new subjects may be recruited to the study and placed on the investigational drug; patients already in the study should be taken off therapy involving the investigational drug unless specifically permitted by FDA in the interest of patient safety.

(b) Grounds for imposition of clinical hold—(1) Clinical hold of a Phase 1 study under an IND. FDA may place a proposed or ongoing Phase 1 investigation on clinical hold if it finds that:

(i) Human subjects are or would be exposed to an unreasonable and significant risk of illness or injury;

(ii) The clinical investigators named in the IND are not qualified by reason of their scientific training and experience to conduct the investigation described in the IND;

(iii) The investigator brochure is misleading, erroneous, or materially incomplete; or

(iv) The IND does not contain sufficient information required under Sec. 312.23 to assess the risks to subjects of the proposed studies.

(2) Clinical hold of a Phase 2 or 3 study under an IND. FDA may place a proposed or ongoing Phase 2 or 3 investigation on clinical hold if it finds that:

(i) Any of the conditions in paragraph (b)(1)(i) through (iv) of this section apply; or

(ii) The plan or protocol for the investigation is clearly deficient in design to meet its stated objectives.

(3) Clinical hold of a treatment IND or treatment protocol.

(i) Proposed use. FDA may place a proposed treatment IND or treatment protocol on clinical hold if it is determined that:

(A) The pertinent criteria in Sec. 312.34(b) for permitting the treatment use to begin are not satisfied; or

(B) The treatment protocol or treatment IND does not contain the information required under Sec. 312.35 (a) or (b) to make the specified determination under Sec. 312.34(b).

(ii) Ongoing use. FDA may place an ongoing treatment protocol or treatment IND on clinical hold if it is determined that:

(A) There becomes available a comparable or satisfactory alternative drug or other therapy to treat that stage of the disease in the intended patient population for which the investigational drug is being used;

(B) The investigational drug is not under investigation in a controlled clinical trial under an IND in effect for the trial and not all controlled clinical trials necessary to support a marketing application have been completed, or a clinical study under the IND has been placed on clinical hold:

(C) The sponsor of the controlled clinical trial is not pursuing marketing approval with due diligence;

(D) If the treatment IND or treatment protocol is intended for a serious disease, there is insufficient evidence of safety and effectiveness to support such use; or

(E) If the treatment protocol or treatment IND was based on an immediately life-threatening disease, the available scientific evidence, taken as a whole, fails to provide a reasonable basis for concluding that the drug:

(1) May be effective for its intended use in its intended population; or

(2) Would not expose the patients to whom the drug is to be administered to an unreasonable and significant additional risk of illness or injury.

(iii) FDA may place a proposed or ongoing treatment IND or treatment protocol on clinical hold if it finds that any of the conditions in paragraph (b)(4)(i) through (b)(4)(viii) of this section apply.

(4) Clinical hold of any study that is not designed to be adequate and well-controlled. FDA may place a proposed or ongoing investigation that is not designed to be adequate and well-controlled on clinical hold if it finds that:

(i) Any of the conditions in paragraph (b)(1) or (b)(2) of this section apply; or

(ii) There is reasonable evidence the investigation that is not designed to be adequate and well-controlled is impeding enrollment in, or otherwise interfering with the conduct or completion of, a study that is designed to be an adequate and well-controlled investigation of the same or another investigational drug; or

(iii) Insufficient quantities of the investigational drug exist to adequately conduct both the investigation that is not designed to be adequate and well-controlled and the investigations that are designed to be adequate and well-controlled; or

(iv) The drug has been studied in one or more adequate and well-controlled investigations that strongly suggest lack of effectiveness; or

(v) Another drug under investigation or approved for the same indication and available to the same patient population has demonstrated a better potential benefit/risk balance; or

(vi) The drug has received marketing approval for the same indication in the same patient population; or

(vii) The sponsor of the study that is designed to be an adequate and well-controlled investigation is not actively pursuing marketing approval of the investigational drug with due diligence; or

(viii) The Commissioner determines that it would not be in the public interest for the study to be conducted or continued. FDA ordinarily intends that clinical holds under paragraphs (b)(4)(ii), (b)(4)(iii) and (b)(4)(v) of this section would only apply to additional enrollment in nonconcurrently controlled trials rather than eliminating continued access to individuals already receiving the investigational drug.

(5) Clinical hold of any investigation involving an exception from informed consent under Sec. 50.24 of this chapter. FDA may place a proposed or ongoing investigation involving an exception from informed consent under Sec. 50.24 of this chapter on clinical hold if it is determined that:

(i) Any of the conditions in paragraphs (b)(1) or (b)(2) of this section apply; or

(ii) The pertinent criteria in Sec. 50.24 of this chapter for such an investigation to begin or continue are not submitted or not satisfied.

(c) Discussion of deficiency. Whenever FDA concludes that a deficiency exists in a clinical investigation that may be grounds for the imposition of clinical hold FDA will, unless patients are exposed to immediate and serious risk, attempt to discuss and satisfactorily resolve the matter with the sponsor before issuing the clinical hold order.

(d) Imposition of clinical hold. The clinical hold order may be made by telephone or other means of rapid communication or in writing. The clinical hold order will identify the studies under the IND to which the hold applies, and will briefly explain the basis for the action. The clinical hold order will be made by or on behalf of the Division Director with responsibility for review of the IND. As soon as possible, and no more than 30 days after imposition of the clinical hold, the Division Director will provide the sponsor a written explanation of the basis for the hold.

(e) Resumption of clinical investigations. If, by the terms of the clinical hold order, resumption of the affected investigation is permitted without prior notification by FDA once a stated correction or modification is made, the investigation may proceed as soon as the correction or modification is made. In all other cases, an investigation may only resume after the Division Director (or the Director's designee) with responsibility for review of the IND has notified the sponsor that the investigation may proceed. In these cases resumption of the affected investigation(s) will be authorized when the sponsor corrects the deficiency(ies) previously cited or otherwise satisfied the agency that the investigation(s) can proceed. Resumption of a study may be authorized by telephone or other means of rapid communication.

(f) Appeal. If the sponsor disagrees with the reasons cited for the clinical hold, the sponsor may request reconsideration of the decision in accordance with Sec. 312.48.

(g) Conversion of IND on clinical hold to inactive status. If all investigations covered by an IND remain on clinical hold for 1 year or more, the IND may be placed on inactive status by FDA under Sec. 312.45.

[52 FR 8831, Mar. 19, 1987, as amended at 52 FR 19477, May 22, 1987; 57 FR 13249, Apr. 15, 1992; 61 FR 51530, Oct. 2, 1996]

Sec. 312.44 Termination.

(a) General. This section describes the procedures under which FDA may terminate an IND. If an IND is terminated, the sponsor shall end all clinical investigations conducted under the IND and recall or otherwise provide for the disposition of all unused supplies of the drug. A termination action may be based on deficiencies in the IND or in the conduct of an investigation under an IND. Except as provided in paragraph (d) of this section, a termination shall be preceded by a proposal to terminate by FDA and an opportunity for the sponsor to respond. FDA will, in general, only initiate an action under this section after first attempting to resolve differences informally or, when appropriate, through the clinical hold procedures described in Sec. 312.42.

(b) Grounds for termination—(1) Phase 1. FDA may propose to terminate an IND during Phase 1 if it finds that:

(i) Human subjects would be exposed to an unreasonable and significant risk of illness or unjury.

(ii) The IND does not contain sufficient information required under Sec. 312.23 to assess the safety to subjects of the clinical investigations.

(iii) The methods, facilities, and controls used for the manufacturing, processing, and packing of the investigational drug are inadequate to establish and maintain appropriate standards of identity, strength, quality, and purity as needed for subject safety.

(iv) The clinical investigations are being conducted in a manner substantially different than that described in the protocols submitted in the IND.

(v) The drug is being promoted or distributed for commercial purposes not justified by the requirements of the investigation or permitted by Sec. 312.7.

(vi) The IND, or any amendment or report to the IND, contains an untrue statement of a material fact or omits material information required by this part.

(vii) The sponsor fails promptly to investigate and inform the Food and Drug Administration and all investigators of serious and unexpected adverse experiences in accordance with Sec. 312.32 or fails to make any other report required under this part.

(viii) The sponsor fails to submit an accurate annual report of the investigations in accordance with Sec. 312.33.

(ix) The sponsor fails to comply with any other applicable requirement of this part, part 50, or part 56.

(x) The IND has remained on inactive status for 5 years or more.

(xi) The sponsor fails to delay a proposed investigation under the IND or to suspend an ongoing investigation that has been placed on clinical hold under Sec. 312.42(b)(4).

(2) Phase 2 or 3. FDA may propose to terminate an IND during Phase 2 or Phase 3 if FDA finds that:

(i) Any of the conditions in paragraphs (b)(1)(i) through (b)(1)(xi) of this section apply; or

(ii) The investigational plan or protocol(s) is not reasonable as a bona fide scientific plan to determine whether or not the drug is safe and effective for use; or

(iii) There is convincing evidence that the drug is not effective for the purpose for which it is being investigated.

(3) FDA may propose to terminate a treatment IND if it finds that:

(i) Any of the conditions in paragraphs (b)(1)(i) through (x) of this section apply; or

(ii) Any of the conditions in Sec. 312.42(b)(3) apply.

(c) Opportunity for sponsor response. (1) If FDA proposes to terminate an IND, FDA will notify the sponsor in writing, and invite correction or explanation within a period of 30 days.

(2) On such notification, the sponsor may provide a written explanation or correction or may request a conference with FDA to provide the requested explanation or correction. If the sponsor does not respond to the notification within the allocated time, the IND shall be terminated.

(3) If the sponsor responds but FDA does not accept the explanation or correction submitted, FDA shall inform the sponsor in writing of the reason for the nonacceptance and provide the sponsor with an opportunity for a regulatory hearing before FDA under part 16 on the question of whether the IND should be terminated. The sponsor's request for a regulatory hearing must be made within 10 days of the sponsor's receipt of FDA's notification of nonacceptance.

(d) Immediate termination of IND. Notwithstanding paragraphs (a) through (c) of this section, if at any time FDA concludes that continuation of the investigation presents an immediate and substantial danger to the health of individuals, the agency shall immediately, by written notice to the sponsor from the Director of the Center for Drug Evaluation and Research or the Director of the Center for Biologics Evaluation and Research, terminate the IND. An IND so terminated is subject to reinstatement by the Director on the basis of additional submissions that eliminate such danger. If an IND is terminated under this paragraph, the agency will afford the sponsor an opportunity for a regulatory hearing under part 16 on the question of whether the IND should be reinstated.

(Collection of information requirements approved by the Office of Management and Budget under control number 0910-0014)

[52 FR 8831, Mar. 19, 1987, as amended at 52 FR 23031, June 17, 1987; 55 FR 11579, Mar. 29, 1990; 57 FR 13249, Apr. 15, 1992]

Sec. 312.45 Inactive status.

(a) If no subjects are entered into clinical studies for a period of 2 years or more under an IND, or if all investigations under an IND remain on clinical hold for 1 year or more, the IND may be placed by FDA on inactive status. This action may be taken by FDA either on request of the sponsor or on FDA's own initiative. If FDA seeks to act on its own initiative under this section, it shall first notify the sponsor in writing of the proposed inactive status. Upon receipt of such notification, the sponsor shall have 30 days to respond as to why the IND should continue to remain active.

(b) If an IND is placed on inactive status, all investigators shall be so notified and all stocks of the drug shall be returned or otherwise disposed of in accordance with Sec. 312.59.

(c) A sponsor is not required to submit annual reports to an IND on inactive status. An inactive IND is, however, still in effect for purposes of the public disclosure of data and information under Sec. 312.130.

(d) A sponsor who intends to resume clinical investigation under an IND placed on inactive status shall submit a protocol amendment under Sec. 312.30 containing the proposed general investigational plan for the coming year and appropriate protocols. If the protocol amendment relies on information previously submitted, the plan shall reference such information. Additional information supporting the proposed investigation, if any, shall be submitted in an information amendment. Notwithstanding the provisions of Sec. 312.30, clinical investigations under an IND on inactive status may only resume (1) 30 days after FDA receives the protocol amendment, unless FDA notifies the sponsor that the investigations described in the amendment are subject to a clinical hold under Sec. 312.42, or (2) on earlier notification by FDA that the clinical investigations described in the protocol amendment may begin.

(e) An IND that remains on inactive status for 5 years or more may be terminated under Sec. 312.44.

(Collection of information requirements approved by the Office of Management and Budget under control number 0910-0014)

[52 FR 8831, Mar. 19, 1987, as amended at 52 FR 23031, June 17, 1987]

Sec. 312.47 Meetings.

(a) General. Meetings between a sponsor and the agency are frequently useful in resolving questions and issues raised during the course of a clinical investigation. FDA encourages such meetings to the extent that they aid in the evaluation of the drug and in the solution of scientific problems concerning the drug, to the extent that FDA's resources permit. The general principle underlying the conduct of such meetings is that there should be free, full, and open communication about any scientific or medical question that may arise during the clinical investigation. These meetings shall be conducted and documented in accordance with part 10.

(b) "End-of-Phase 2" meetings and meetings held before submission of a marketing application. At specific times during the drug investigation process, meetings between FDA and a sponsor can be especially helpful in minimizing wasteful expenditures of time and money and thus in speeding the drug development and evaluation process. In particular, FDA has found that meetings at the end of Phase 2 of an investigation (end-of-Phase 2 meetings) are of considerable assistance in planning later studies and that meetings held near completion of Phase 3 and before submission of a marketing application ("pre-NDA" meetings) are helpful in developing methods of presentation and submission of data in the marketing application that facilitate review and allow timely FDA response.(1) End-of-Phase 2 meetings—(i) Purpose. The purpose of an end-of-Phase 2 meeting is to determine the safety of proceeding to Phase 3, to evaluate the Phase 3 plan and protocols, and to identify any additional information necessary to support a marketing application for the uses under investigation.

(ii) Eligibility for meeting. While the end-of-Phase 2 meeting is designed primarily for IND's involving new molecular entities or major new uses of marketed drugs, a sponsor of any IND may request and obtain an end-of-Phase 2 meeting.

(iii) Timing. To be most useful to the sponsor, end-of-Phase 2 meetings should be held before major commitments of effort and resources to specific Phase 3 tests are made. The scheduling of an end-of-Phase 2 meeting is not, however, intended to delay the transition of an investigation from Phase 2 to Phase 3.

(iv) Advance information. At least 1 month in advance of an end-of-Phase 2 meeting, the sponsor should submit background information on the sponsor's plan for Phase 3, including summaries of the Phase 1 and 2 investigations, the specific protocols for Phase 3 clinical studies, plans for any additional nonclinical studies, and, if available, tentative labeling for the drug. The recommended contents of such a submission are described more fully in FDA Staff Manual Guide 4850.7 that is publicly available under FDA's public information regulations in part 20.

(v) Conduct of meeting. Arrangements for an end-of-Phase 2 meeting are to be made with the division in FDA's Center for Drug Evaluation and Research or the Center for Biologics Evaluation and Research which is responsible for review of the IND. The meeting will be scheduled by FDA at a time convenient to both FDA and the sponsor. Both the sponsor and FDA may bring consultants to the meeting. The meeting should be directed primarily at establishing agreement between FDA and the sponsor of the overall plan for Phase 3 and the objectives and design of particular studies. The adequacy of technical information to support Phase 3 studies and/or a marketing application may also be discussed. Agreements reached at the meeting on these matters will be recorded in minutes of the conference that will be taken by FDA in accordance with Sec. 10.65 and provided to the sponsor. The minutes along with any other written material provided to the sponsor will serve as a permanent record of any agreements reached. Barring a significant scientific development that requires otherwise, studies conducted in accordance with the agreement shall be presumed to be sufficient in objective and design for the purpose of obtaining marketing approval for the drug.

(2) "Pre-NDA" meetings. FDA has found that delays associated with the initial review of a marketing application may be reduced by exchanges of information about a proposed marketing application. The primary purpose of this kind of exchange is to uncover any major unresolved problems, to identify those studies that the sponsor is relying on as adequate and well-controlled to establish the drug's effectiveness, to acquaint FDA reviewers with the general information to be submitted in the marketing application (including technical information), to discuss appropriate methods for statistical analysis of the data, and to discuss the best approach to the presentation and formatting of data in the marketing application. Arrangements for such a meeting are to be initiated by the sponsor with the division responsible for review of the IND. To permit FDA to provide the sponsor with the most useful advice on preparing a marketing application, the sponsor should submit to FDA's reviewing division at least 1 month in advance of the meeting the following information:

(i) A brief summary of the clinical studies to be submitted in the application.

(ii) A proposed format for organizing the submission, including methods for presenting the data.

(iii) Any other information for discussion at the meeting.

(Collection of information requirements approved by the Office of Management and Budget under control number 0910-0014)

[52 FR 8831, Mar. 19, 1987, as amended at 52 FR 23031, June 17, 1987; 55 FR 11580, Mar. 29, 1990]

Sec. 312.48 Dispute resolution.

(a) General. The Food and Drug Administration is committed to resolving differences between sponsors and FDA reviewing divisions with respect to requirements for IND's as quickly and amicably as possible through the cooperative exchange of information and views.

(b) Administrative and procedural issues. When administrative or procedural disputes arise, the sponsor should first attempt to resolve the matter with the division in FDA's Center for Drug Evaluation and Research or Center for Biologics Evaluation and Research which is responsible for review of the IND, beginning with the consumer safety officer assigned to the application. If the dispute is not resolved, the sponsor may raise the matter with the person designated as ombudsman, whose function shall be to investigate what has happened and to facilitate a timely and equitable resolution. Appropriate issues to raise with the ombudsman include resolving difficulties in scheduling meetings and obtaining timely replies to inquiries. Further details on this procedure are contained in FDA Staff Manual Guide 4820.7 that is publicly available under FDA's public information regulations in part 20.

(c) Scientific and medical disputes. (1) When scientific or medical disputes arise during the drug investigation process, sponsors should discuss the matter directly with the responsible reviewing officials. If necessary, sponsors may request a meeting with the appropriate reviewing officials and management representatives in order to seek a resolution. Requests for such meetings shall be directed to the director of the division in FDA's Center for Drug Evaluation and Research or Center for Biologics Evaluation and Research which is responsible for review of the IND. FDA will make every attempt to grant requests for meetings that involve important issues and that can be scheduled at mutually convenient times.

(2) The "end-of-Phase 2" and "pre-NDA" meetings described in Sec. 312.47(b) will also provide a timely forum for discussing and resolving scientific and medical issues on which the sponsor disagrees with the agency.

(3) In requesting a meeting designed to resolve a scientific or medical dispute, applicants may suggest that FDA seek the advice of outside experts, in which case FDA may, in its discretion, invite to the meeting one or more of its advisory committee members or other consultants, as designated by the agency. Applicants may rely on, and may bring to any meeting, their own consultants. For major scientific and medical policy issues not resolved by informal meetings, FDA may refer the matter to one of its standing advisory committees for its consideration and recommendations.

[52 FR 8831, Mar. 19, 1987, as amended at 55 FR 11580, Mar. 29, 1990]

Subpart D—Responsibilities of Sponsors and Investigators

Sec. 312.50 General responsibilities of sponsors.

Sponsors are responsible for selecting qualified investigators, providing them with the information they need to conduct an investigation properly, ensuring proper monitoring of the investigation(s), ensuring that the investigation(s) is conducted in accordance with the general investigational plan and protocols contained in the IND, maintaining an effective IND with respect to the investigations, and ensuring that FDA and all participating investigators are promptly informed of significant new adverse effects or risks with respect to the drug. Additional specific responsibilities of sponsors are described elsewhere in this part.

Sec. 312.52 Transfer of obligations to a contract research organization.

(a) A sponsor may transfer responsibility for any or all of the obligations set forth in this part to a contract research organization. Any such transfer shall be described in writing. If not all obligations are transferred, the writing is required to describe each of the obligations being assumed by the contract research organization. If all obligations are transferred, a general statement that all obligations have been transferred is acceptable. Any obligation not covered by the written description shall be deemed not to have been transferred.

(b) A contract research organization that assumes any obligation of a sponsor shall comply with the specific regulations in this chapter applicable to this obligation and shall be subject to the same regulatory action as a sponsor for failure to comply with any obligation assumed under these regulations. Thus, all references to "sponsor" in this part apply to a contract research organization to the extent that it assumes one or more obligations of the sponsor.

Sec. 312.53 Selecting investigators and monitors.

(a) Selecting investigators. A sponsor shall select only investigators qualified by training and experience as appropriate experts to investigate the drug.

(b) Control of drug. A sponsor shall ship investigational new drugs only to investigators participating in the investigation.

(c) Obtaining information from the investigator. Before permitting an investigator to begin participation in an investigation, the sponsor shall obtain the following:

(1) A signed investigator statement (Form FDA-1572) containing:

(i) The name and address of the investigator;

(ii) The name and code number, if any, of the protocol(s) in the IND identifying the study(ies) to be conducted by the investigator;

(iii) The name and address of any medical school, hospital, or other research facility where the clinical investigation(s) will be conducted;

(iv) The name and address of any clinical laboratory facilities to be used in the study;

(v) The name and address of the IRB that is responsible for review and approval of the study(ies);

(vi) A commitment by the investigator that he or she:

(a) Will conduct the study(ies) in accordance with the relevant, current protocol(s) and will only make changes in a protocol after notifying the sponsor, except when necessary to protect the safety, the rights, or welfare of subjects;

(b) Will comply with all requirements regarding the obligations of clinical investigators and all other pertinent requirements in this part;

(c) Will personally conduct or supervise the described investigation(s);

(d) Will inform any potential subjects that the drugs are being used for investigational purposes and will ensure that the requirements relating to obtaining informed consent (21 CFR part 50) and institutional review board review and approval (21 CFR part 56) are met;

(e) Will report to the sponsor adverse experiences that occur in the course of the investigation(s) in accordance with Sec. 312.64;

(f) Has read and understands the information in the investigator's brochure, including the potential risks and side effects of the drug; and

(g) Will ensure that all associates, colleagues, and employees assisting in the conduct of the study(ies) are informed about their obligations in meeting the above commitments.

(vii) A commitment by the investigator that, for an investigation subject to an institutional review requirement under part 56, an IRB that complies with the requirements of that part will be responsible for the initial and continuing review and approval of the clinical investigation and that the investigator will promptly report to the IRB all changes in the research activity and all unanticipated problems involving risks to human subjects or others, and will not make any changes in the research without IRB approval, except where necessary to eliminate apparent immediate hazards to the human subjects.

(viii) A list of the names of the subinvestigators (e.g., research fellows, residents) who will be assisting the investigator in the conduct of the investigation(s).

(2) Curriculum vitae. A curriculum vitae or other statement of qualifications of the investigator showing the education, training, and experience that qualifies the investigator as an expert in the clinical investigation of the drug for the use under investigation.

(3) Clinical protocol. (i) For Phase 1 investigations, a general outline of the planned investigation including the estimated duration of the study and the maximum number of subjects that will be involved.

(ii) For Phase 2 or 3 investigations, an outline of the study protocol including an approximation of the number of subjects to be treated with the drug and the number to be employed as controls, if any; the clinical uses to be investigated; characteristics of subjects by age, sex, and condition; the kind of clinical observations and laboratory tests to be conducted; the estimated duration of the study; and copies or a description of case report forms to be used.

(4) Financial disclosure information. Sufficient accurate financial information to allow the sponsor to submit complete and accurate certification or disclosure statements required under part 54 of this chapter. The sponsor shall obtain a commitment from the clinical investigator to promptly update this information if any relevant changes occur during the course of the investigation and for 1 year following the completion of the study.

(d) Selecting monitors. A sponsor shall select a monitor qualified by training and experience to monitor the progress of the investigation.

(Collection of information requirements approved by the Office of Management and Budget under control number 0910-0014)

[52 FR 8831, Mar. 19, 1987, as amended at 52 FR 23031, June 17, 1987; 61 FR 57280, Nov. 5, 1996; 63 FR 5252, Feb. 2, 1998]

Effective Date Note: At 63 FR 5252, Feb. 2, 1998, Sec. 312.53 was amended by adding new paragraph (c)(4), effective Feb. 2, 1999.

Sec. 312.54 Emergency research under Sec. 50.24 of this chapter.

(a) The sponsor shall monitor the progress of all investigations involving an exception from informed consent under Sec. 50.24 of this chapter. When the sponsor receives from the IRB information concerning the public disclosures required by Sec. 50.24(a)(7)(ii) and (a)(7)(iii) of this chapter, the sponsor promptly shall submit to the IND file and to Docket Number 95S-0158 in the Dockets Management Branch (HFA-305), Food and Drug Administration, 12420 Parklawn Dr., rm. 1-23, Rockville, MD 20857, copies of the information that was disclosed, identified by the IND number.

(b) The sponsor also shall monitor such investigations to identify when an IRB determines that it cannot approve the research because it does not meet the criteria in the exception in Sec. 50.24(a) of this chapter or because of other relevant ethical concerns. The sponsor promptly shall provide this information in writing to FDA, investigators who are asked to participate in this or a substantially equivalent clinical investigation, and other IRB's that are asked to review this or a substantially equivalent investigation.

[61 FR 51530, Oct. 2, 1996]

Sec. 312.55 Informing investigators.

(a) Before the investigation begins, a sponsor (other than a sponsor-investigator) shall give each participating clinical investigator an investigator brochure containing the information described in Sec. 312.23(a)(5).

(b) The sponsor shall, as the overall investigation proceeds, keep each participating investigator informed of new observations discovered by or reported to the sponsor on the drug, particularly with respect to adverse effects and safe use. Such information may be distributed to investigators by means of periodically revised investigator brochures, reprints or published studies, reports or letters to clinical investigators, or other appropriate means.Important safety information is required to be relayed to investigators in accordance with Sec. 312.32.

(Collection of information requirements approved by the Office of Management and Budget under control number 0910-0014)

[52 FR 8831, Mar. 19, 1987, as amended at 52 FR 23031, June 17, 1987]

Sec. 312.56 Review of ongoing investigations.

(a) The sponsor shall monitor the progress of all clinical investigations being conducted under its IND.

(b) A sponsor who discovers that an investigator is not complying with the signed agreement (Form FDA-1572), the general investigational plan, or the requirements of this part or other applicable parts shall promptly either secure compliance or discontinue shipments of the investigational new drug to the investigator and end the investigator's participation in the investigation. If the investigator's participation in the investigation is ended, the sponsor shall require that the investigator dispose of or return the investigational drug in accordance with the requirements of Sec. 312.59 and shall notify FDA.

(c) The sponsor shall review and evaluate the evidence relating to the safety and effectiveness of the drug as it is obtained from the investigator. The sponsors shall make such reports to FDA regarding information relevant to the safety of the drug as are required under Sec. 312.32. The sponsor shall make annual reports on the progress of the investigation in accordance with Sec. 312.33.

(d) A sponsor who determines that its investigational drug presents an unreasonable and significant risk to subjects shall discontinue those investigations that present the risk, notify FDA, all institutional review boards, and all investigators who have at any time participated in the investigation of the discontinuance, assure the disposition of all stocks of the drug outstanding as required by Sec. 312.59, and furnish FDA with a full report of the sponsor's actions. The sponsor shall discontinue the investigation as soon as possible, and in no event later than 5 working days after making the determination that the investigation should be discontinued. Upon request, FDA will confer with a sponsor on the need to discontinue an investigation.

(Collection of information requirements approved by the Office of Management and Budget under control number 0910-0014)

[52 FR 8831, Mar. 19, 1987, as amended at 52 FR 23031, June 17, 1987]

Sec. 312.57 Recordkeeping and record retention.

(a) A sponsor shall maintain adequate records showing the receipt, shipment, or other disposition of the investigational drug. These records are required to include, as appropriate, the name of the investigator to whom the drug is shipped, and the date, quantity, and batch or code mark of each such shipment.

(b) A sponsor shall maintain complete and accurate records showing any financial interest in Sec. 54.4(a)(3)(i), (a)(3)(ii), (a)(3)(iii), and (a)(3)(iv) of this chapter paid to clinical investigators by the sponsor of the covered study. A sponsor shall also maintain complete and accurate records concerning all other financial interests of investigators subject to part 54 of this chapter.

(c) A sponsor shall retain the records and reports required by this part for 2 years after a marketing application is approved for the drug; or, if an application is not approved for the drug, until 2 years after shipment and delivery of the drug for investigational use is discontinued and FDA has been so notified.

(d) A sponsor shall retain reserve samples of any test article and reference standard identified in, and used in any of the bioequivalence or bioavailability studies described in, Sec. 320.38 or Sec. 320.63 of this chapter, and release the reserve samples to FDA upon request, in accordance with, and for the period specified in Sec. 320.38.

(Collection of information requirements approved by the Office of Management and Budget under control number 0910-0014)

[52 FR 8831, Mar. 19, 1987, as amended at 52 FR 23031, June 17, 1987; 58 FR 25926, Apr. 28, 1993; 63 FR 5252, Feb. 2, 1998]

Effective Date Note: At 63 FR 5252, Feb. 2, 1998, Sec. 312.57 was amended by redesignating paragraphs (b) and (c) as paragraphs (c) and (d) and by adding a new paragraph (b), effective Feb. 2, 1999.

Sec. 312.58 Inspection of sponsor's records and reports.

(a) FDA inspection. A sponsor shall upon request from any properly authorized officer or employee of the Food and Drug Administration, at reasonable times, permit such officer or employee to have access to and copy and verify any records and reports relating to a clinical investigation conducted under this part. Upon written request by FDA, the sponsor shall submit the records or reports (or copies of them) to FDA. The sponsor shall discontinue shipments of the drug to any investigator who has failed to maintain or make available records or reports of the investigation as required by this part.

(b) Controlled substances. If an investigational new drug is a substance listed in any schedule of the Controlled Substances Act (21 U.S.C. 801; 21 CFR part 1308), records concerning shipment, delivery, receipt, and disposition of the drug, which are required to be kept under this part or other applicable parts of this chapter shall, upon the request of a properly authorized employee of the Drug Enforcement Administration of the U.S. Department of Justice, be made available by the investigator or sponsor to whom the request is made, for inspection and copying. In addition, the sponsor shall assure that adequate precautions are taken, including storage of the investigational drug in a securely locked, substantially constructed cabinet, or other securely locked, substantially constructed enclosure, access to which is limited, to prevent theft or diversion of the substance into illegal channels of distribution.

Sec. 312.59 Disposition of unused supply of investigational drug.

The sponsor shall assure the return of all unused supplies of the investigational drug from each individual investigator whose participation in the investigation is discontinued or terminated. The sponsor may authorize alternative disposition of unused supplies of the investigational drug provided this alternative disposition does not expose humans to risks from the drug. The sponsor shall maintain written records of any disposition of the drug in accordance with Sec. 312.57.

(Collection of information requirements approved by the Office of Management and Budget under control number 0910-0014)

[52 FR 8831, Mar. 19, 1987, as amended at 52 FR 23031, June 17, 1987]

Sec. 312.60 General responsibilities of investigators.

An investigator is responsible for ensuring that an investigation is conducted according to the signed investigator statement, the investigational plan, and applicable regulations; for protecting the rights, safety, and welfare of subjects under the investigator's care; and for the control of drugs under investigation. An investigator shall, in accordance with the provisions of part 50 of this chapter, obtain the informed consent of each human subject to whom the drug is administered, except as provided in Secs. 50.23 or 50.24 of this chapter. Additional specific responsibilities of clinical investigators are set forth in this part and in parts 50 and 56 of this chapter.

[52 FR 8831, Mar. 19, 1987, as amended at 61 FR 51530, Oct. 2, 1996]

Sec. 312.61 Control of the investigational drug.

An investigator shall administer the drug only to subjects under the investigator's personal supervision or under the supervision of a subinvestigator responsible to the investigator. The investigator shall not supply the investigational drug to any person not authorized under this part to receive it.

Sec. 312.62 Investigator recordkeeping and record retention.

(a) Disposition of drug. An investigator is required to maintain adequate records of the disposition of the drug, including dates, quantity, and use by subjects. If the investigation is terminated, suspended, discontinued, or completed, the investigator shall return the unused supplies of the drug to the sponsor, or otherwise provide for disposition of the unused supplies of the drug under Sec. 312.59.

(b) Case histories. An investigator is required to prepare and maintain adequate and accurate case histories that record all observations and other data pertinent to the investigation on each individual administered the investigational drug or employed as a control in the investigation. Case histories include the case report forms and supporting data including, for example, signed and dated consent forms and medical records including, for example, progress notes of the physician, the individual's hospital chart(s), and the nurses' notes. The case history for each individual shall document that informed consent was obtained prior to participation in the study.

(c) Record retention. An investigator shall retain records required to be maintained under this part for a period of 2 years following the date a marketing application is approved for the drug for the indication for which it is being investigated; or, if no application is to be filed or if the application is not approved for such indication, until 2 years after the investigation is discontinued and FDA is notified.

(Collection of information requirements approved by the Office of Management and Budget under control number 0910-0014)

[52 FR 8831, Mar. 19, 1987, as amended at 52 FR 23031, June 17, 1987; 61 FR 57280, Nov. 5, 1996]

Sec. 312.64 Investigator reports.

(a) Progress reports. The investigator shall furnish all reports to the sponsor of the drug who is responsible for collecting and evaluating the results obtained. The sponsor is required under Sec. 312.33 to submit annual reports to FDA on the progress of the clinical investigations.

(b) Safety reports. An investigator shall promptly report to the sponsor any adverse effect that may reasonably be regarded as caused by, or probably caused by, the drug. If the adverse effect is alarming, the investigator shall report the adverse effect immediately.

(c) Final report. An investigator shall provide the sponsor with an adequate report shortly after completion of the investigator's participation in the investigation.

(d) Financial disclosure reports. The clinical investigator shall provide the sponsor with sufficient accurate financial information to allow an applicant to submit complete and accurate certification or disclosure statements as required under part 54 of this chapter. The clinical investigator shall promptly update this information if any relevant changes occur during the course of the investigation and for 1 year following the completion of the study.

(Collection of information requirements approved by the Office of Management and Budget under control number 0910-0014)

[52 FR 8831, Mar. 19, 1987, as amended at 52 FR 23031, June 17, 1987; 63 FR 5252, Feb. 2, 1998]

Effective Date Note: At 63 FR 5252, Feb. 2, 1998, Sec. 312.64 was amended by adding new paragraph (d), effective Feb. 2, 1999.

Sec. 312.66 Assurance of IRB review.

An investigator shall assure that an IRB that complies with the requirements set forth in part 56 will be responsible for the initial and continuing review and approval of the proposed clinical study. The investigator shall also assure that he or she will promptly report to the IRB all changes in the research activity and all unanticipated problems involving risk to human subjects or others, and that he or she will not make any changes in the research without IRB approval, except where necessary to eliminate apparent immediate hazards to human subjects.

(Collection of information requirements approved by the Office of Management and Budget under control number 0910-0014)

[52 FR 8831, Mar. 19, 1987, as amended at 52 FR 23031, June 17, 1987]

Sec. 312.68 Inspection of investigator's records and reports.

An investigator shall upon request from any properly authorized officer or employee of FDA, at reasonable times, permit such officer or employee to have access to, and copy and verify any records or reports made by the investigator pursuant to Sec. 312.62. The investigator is not required to divulge subject names unless the records of particular individuals require a more detailed study of the cases, or unless there is reason to believe that the records do not represent actual case studies, or do not represent actual results obtained.

Sec. 312.69 Handling of controlled substances.

If the investigational drug is subject to the Controlled Substances Act, the investigator shall take adequate precautions, including storage of the investigational drug in a securely locked, substantially constructed cabinet, or other securely locked, substantially constructed enclosure, access to which is limited, to prevent theft or diversion of the substance into illegal channels of distribution.

Sec. 312.70 Disqualification of a clinical investigator.

(a) If FDA has information indicating that an investigator (including a sponsor-investigator) has repeatedly or deliberately failed to comply with the requirements of this part, part 50, or part 56 of this chapter, or has submitted to FDA or to the sponsor false information in any required report, the Center for Drug Evaluation and Research or the Center for Biologics Evaluation and Research will furnish the investigator written notice of the matter complained of and offer the investigator an opportunity to explain the matter in writing, or, at the option of the investigator, in an informal conference. If an explanation is offered but not accepted by the Center for Drug Evaluation and Research or the Center for Biologics

Evaluation and Research, the investigator will be given an opportunity for a regulatory hearing under part 16 on the question of whether the investigator is entitled to receive investigational new drugs.

(b) After evaluating all available information, including any explanation presented by the investigator, if the Commissioner determines that the investigator has repeatedly or deliberately failed to comply with the requirements of this part, part 50, or part 56 of this chapter, or has deliberately or repeatedly submitted false information to FDA or to the sponsor in any required report, the Commissioner will notify the investigator and the sponsor of any investigation in which the investigator has been named as a participant that the investigator is not entitled to receive investigational drugs. The notification will provide a statement of basis for such determination.

(c) Each IND and each approved application submitted under part 314 containing data reported by an investigator who has been determined to be ineligible to receive investigational drugs will be examined to determine whether the investigator has submitted unreliable data that are essential to the continuation of the investigation or essential to the approval of any marketing application.

(d) If the Commissioner determines, after the unreliable data submitted by the investigator are eliminated from consideration, that the data remaining are inadequate to support a conclusion that it is reasonably safe to continue the investigation, the Commissioner will notify the sponsor who shall have an opportunity for a regulatory hearing under part 16. If a danger to the public health exists, however, the Commissioner shall terminate the IND immediately and notify the sponsor of the determination. In such case, the sponsor shall have an opportunity for a regulatory hearing before FDA under part 16 on the question of whether the IND should be reinstated.

(e) If the Commissioner determines, after the unreliable data submitted by the investigator are eliminated from consideration, that the continued approval of the drug product for which the data were submitted cannot be justified, the Commissioner will proceed to withdraw approval of the drug product in accordance with the applicable provisions of the act.

(f) An investigator who has been determined to be ineligible to receive investigational drugs may be reinstated as eligible when the Commissioner determines that the investigator has presented adequate assurances that the investigator will employ investigational drugs solely in compliance with the provisions of this part and of parts 50 and 56.

(Collection of information requirements approved by the Office of Management and Budget under control number 0910-0014)

[52 FR 8831, Mar. 19, 1987, as amended at 52 FR 23031, June 17, 1987; 55 FR 11580, Mar. 29, 1990; 62 FR 46876, Sept. 5, 1997]

Subpart E—Drugs Intended to Treat Life-threatening and Severely-debilitating Illnesses

Sec. 312.80 Purpose.

Authority: Secs. 501, 502, 503, 505, 506, 507, 701, 52 Stat. 1049-1053 as amended, 1055-1056 as amended, 55 Stat. 851, 59 Stat. 463 as amended (21 U.S.C. 351, 352, 353, 355, 356, 357, 371); sec. 351, 58 Stat. 702 as amended (42 U.S.C. 262); 21 CFR 5.10, 5.11.

Source: 53 FR 41523, Oct. 21, 1988, unless otherwise noted.

The purpose of this section is to establish procedures designed to expedite the development, evaluation, and marketing of new therapies intended to treat persons with life-threatening and severely-debilitating illnesses, especially where no satisfactory alternative therapy exists. As stated Sec. 314.105(c) of this chapter, while the statutory standards of safety and effectiveness apply to all drugs, the many kinds of drugs that are subject to them, and the wide range of uses for those drugs, demand flexibility in applying the standards. The Food and Drug Administration (FDA) has determined that it is appropriate to exercise the broadest flexibility in applying the statutory standards, while preserving appropriate guarantees for safety and effectiveness. These procedures reflect the recognition that physicians and patients are generally willing to accept greater risks or side effects from products that treat life-threatening and severely-debilitating illnesses, than they would accept from products that treat less serious illnesses. These procedures also reflect the recognition that the benefits of the drug need to be evaluated in light of the severity of the disease being treated. The procedure outlined in this section should be interpreted consistent with that purpose.

Sec. 312.81 Scope.

This section applies to new drug, antibiotic, and biological products that are being studied for their safety and effectiveness in treating life-threatening or severely-debilitating diseases.

(a) For purposes of this section, the term "life-threatening" means:

(1) Diseases or conditions where the likelihood of death is high unless the course of the disease is interrupted; and

(2) Diseases or conditions with potentially fatal outcomes, where the end point of clinical trial analysis is survival.

(b) For purposes of this section, the term "severely debilitating" means diseases or conditions that cause major irreversible morbidity.

(c) Sponsors are encouraged to consult with FDA on the applicability of these procedures to specific products.

Sec. 312.82 Early consultation.

For products intended to treat life-threatening or severely-debilitating illnesses, sponsors may request to meet with FDA-reviewing officials early in the drug development process to review and reach agreement on the design of necessary preclinical and clinical studies. Where appropriate, FDA will invite to such meetings one or more outside expert scientific consultants or advisory committee members. To the extent FDA resources permit, agency reviewing officials will honor requests for such meetings.

(a) Pre-investigational new drug (IND) meetings. Prior to the submission of the initial IND, the sponsor may request a meeting with FDA-reviewing officials. The primary purpose of this meeting is to review and reach agreement on the design of animal studies needed to initiate human testing. The meeting may also provide an opportunity for discussing the scope and design of phase 1 testing, and the best approach for presentation and formatting of data in the IND.

(b) End-of-phase 1 meetings. When data from phase 1 clinical testing are available, the sponsor may again request a meeting with FDA-reviewing officials. The primary purpose of this meeting is to review and reach agreement on the design of phase 2 controlled clinical trials, with the goal that such testing will be adequate to provide sufficient data on the drug's safety and effectiveness to support a decision on its approvability for marketing. The procedures outlined in Sec. 312.47(b)(1) with respect to end-of-phase 2 conferences, including documentation of agreements reached, would also be used for end-of-phase 1 meetings.

Sec. 312.83 Treatment protocols.

If the preliminary analysis of phase 2 test results appears promising, FDA may ask the sponsor to submit a treatment protocol to be reviewed under the procedures and criteria listed in Secs. 312.34 and 312.35. Such a treatment protocol, if requested and granted, would normally remain in effect while the complete data necessary for a marketing application are being assembled by the sponsor and reviewed by FDA (unless grounds exist for clinical hold of ongoing protocols, as provided in Sec. 312.42(b)(3)(ii)).

Sec. 312.84 Risk-benefit analysis in review of marketing applications for drugs to treat life-threatening and severely-debilitating illnesses.

(a) FDA's application of the statutory standards for marketing approval shall recognize the need for a medical risk-benefit judgment in making the final decision on approvability. As part of this evaluation, consistent with the statement of purpose in Sec. 312.80, FDA will consider whether the benefits of the drug outweigh the known and potential risks of the drug and the need to answer remaining questions about risks and benefits of the drug, taking into consideration the severity of the disease and the absence of satisfactory alternative therapy.

(b) In making decisions on whether to grant marketing approval for products that have been the subject of an end-of-phase 1 meeting under Sec. 312.82, FDA will usually seek the advice of outside expert scientific consultants or advisory committees. Upon the filing of such a marketing application under Sec. 314.101 or part 601 of this chapter, FDA will notify the members of the relevant standing advisory committee of the application's filing and its availability for review.

(c) If FDA concludes that the data presented are not sufficient for marketing approval, FDA will issue (for a drug) a not approvable letter pursuant to Sec. 314.120 of this chapter, or (for a biologic) a deficiencies letter consistent with the biological product licensing procedures. Such letter, in describing the deficiencies in the application, will address why the results of the research design agreed to under Sec. 312.82, or in subsequent meetings, have not provided sufficient evidence for marketing approval. Such letter will also describe any recommendations made by the advisory committee regarding the application.

(d) Marketing applications submitted under the procedures contained in this section will be subject to the requirements and procedures contained in part 314 or part 600 of this chapter, as well as those in this subpart.

Sec. 312.85 Phase 4 studies.

Concurrent with marketing approval, FDA may seek agreement from the sponsor to conduct certain postmarketing (phase 4) studies to delineate additional information about the drug's risks, benefits, and optimal use. These studies could include, but would not be limited to, studying different doses or schedules of administration than were used in phase 2 studies, use of the drug in other patient populations or other stages of the disease, or use of the drug over a longer period of time.

Sec. 312.86 Focused FDA regulatory research.

At the discretion of the agency, FDA may undertake focused regulatory research on critical rate-limiting aspects of the preclinical, chemical/manufacturing, and clinical phases of drug development and evaluation. When initiated, FDA will undertake such research efforts as a means for meeting a public health need in facilitating the development of therapies to treat life-threatening or severely debilitating illnesses.

Sec. 312.87 Active monitoring of conduct and evaluation of clinical trials.

For drugs covered under this section, the Commissioner and other agency officials will monitor the progress of the conduct and evaluation of clinical trials and be involved in facilitating their appropriate progress.

Sec. 312.88 Safeguards for patient safety.

All of the safeguards incorporated within parts 50, 56, 312, 314, and 600 of this chapter designed to ensure the safety of clinical testing and the safety of products following marketing approval apply to drugs covered by this section. This includes the requirements for informed consent (part 50 of this chapter) and institutional review boards (part 56 of this chapter). These safeguards further include the review of animal studies prior to initial human testing (Sec. 312.23), and the monitoring of adverse drug experiences through the requirements of IND safety reports (Sec. 312.32), safety update reports during agency review of a marketing application (Sec. 314.50 of this chapter), and postmarketing adverse reaction reporting (Sec. 314.80 of this chapter).

Sec. 312.110 Import and export requirements.

(a) Imports. An investigational new drug offered for import into the United States complies with the requirements of this part if it is subject to an IND that is in effect for it under Sec. 312.40 and: (1) The consignee in the United States is the sponsor of the IND; (2) the consignee is a qualified investigator named in the IND; or (3) the consignee is the domestic agent of a foreign sponsor, is responsible for the control and distribution of the investigational drug, and the IND identifies the consignee and describes what, if any, actions the consignee will take with respect to the investigational drug.

(b) Exports. An investigational new drug intended for export from the United States complies with the requirements of this part as follows:

(1) If an IND is in effect for the drug under Sec. 312.40 and each person who receives the drug is an investigator named in the application; or

(2) If FDA authorizes shipment of the drug for use in a clinical investigation. Authorization may be obtained as follows:

(i) Through submission to the International Affairs Staff (HFY-50), Associate Commissioner for Health Affairs, Food and Drug Administration, 5600 Fishers Lane, Rockville, MD 20857, of a written request from the person that seeks to export the drug. A request must provide adequate information about the drug to satisfy FDA that the drug is appropriate for the proposed investigational use in humans, that the drug will be used for investigational purposes only, and that the drug may be legally used by that consignee in the importing country for the proposed investigational use. The request shall specify the quantity of the drug to be shipped per shipment and the frequency of expected shipments. If FDA authorizes exportation under this paragraph, the agency shall concurrently notify the government of the importing country of such authorization.

(ii) Through submission to the International Affairs Staff (HFY-50), Associate Commissioner for Health Affairs, Food and Drug Administration, 5600 Fishers Lane, Rockville, MD 20857, of a formal request from an authorized official of the government of the country to which the drug is proposed to be shipped. A request must specify that the foreign government has adequate information about the drug and the proposed investigational use, that the drug will be used for investigational purposes only, and that the foreign government is satisfied that the drug may legally be used by the intended consignee in that country. Such a request shall specify the quantity of drug to be shipped per shipment and the frequency of expected shipments.

(iii) Authorization to export an investigational drug under paragraph (b)(2)(i) or (ii) of this section may be revoked by FDA if the agency finds that the conditions underlying its authorization are not longer met.

(3) This paragraph applies only where the drug is to be used for the purpose of clinical investigation.

(4) This paragraph does not apply to the export of an antibiotic drug product shipped in accordance with the provisions of section 801(d) of the act.

(5) This paragraph does not apply to the export of new drugs (including biological products) approved for export under section 802 of the act or section 351(h)(1)(A) of the Public Health Service Act.

(Collection of information requirements approved by the Office of Management and Budget under control number 0910-0014)

[52 FR 8831, Mar. 19, 1987, as amended at 52 FR 23031, June 17, 1987]

Subpart F—Miscellaneous

Sec. 312.120 Foreign clinical studies not conducted under an IND.

(a) Introduction. This section describes the criteria for acceptance by FDA of foreign clinical studies not conducted under an IND. In general, FDA accepts such studies provided they are well designed, well conducted, performed by qualified investigators, and conducted in accordance with ethical principles acceptable to the world community. Studies meeting these criteria may be utilized to support clinical investigations in the United States and/or marketing approval. Marketing approval of a new drug or antibiotic drug based solely on foreign clinical data is governed by Sec. 314.106.

(b) Data submissions. A sponsor who wishes to rely on a foreign clinical study to support an IND or to support an application for marketing approval shall submit to FDA the following information:

(1) A description of the investigator's qualifications;

(2) A description of the research facilities;

(3) A detailed summary of the protocol and results of the study, and, should FDA request, case records maintained by the investigator or additional background data such as hospital or other institutional records;

(4) A description of the drug substance and drug product used in the study, including a description of components, formulation, specifications, and bioavailability of the specific drug product used in the clinical study, if available; and

(5) If the study is intended to support the effectiveness of a drug product, information showing that the study is adequate and well controlled under Sec. 314.126.

(c) Conformance with ethical principles. (1) Foreign clinical research is required to have been conducted in accordance with the ethical principles stated in the "Declaration of Helsinki" (see paragraph (c)(4) of this section) or the laws and regulations of the country in which the research was conducted, whichever represents the greater protection of the individual.

(2) For each foreign clinical study submitted under this section, the sponsor shall explain how the research conformed to the ethical principles contained in the "Declaration of Helsinki" or the foreign country's standards, whichever were used. If the foreign country's standards were used, the sponsor shall explain in detail how those standards differ from the "Declaration of Helsinki" and how they offer greater protection.

(3) When the research has been approved by an independent review committee, the sponsor shall submit to FDA documentation of such review and approval, including the names and qualifications of the members of the committee. In this regard, a "review committee" means a committee composed of scientists and, where practicable, individuals who are otherwise qualified (e.g., other health professionals or laymen). The investigator may not vote on any aspect of the review of his or her protocol by a review committee.

(4) The "Declaration of Helsinki" states as follows:

Recommendations Guiding Physicians in Biomedical Research Involving Human Subjects

Introduction

It is the mission of the physician to safeguard the health of the people. His or her knowledge and conscience are dedicated to the fulfillment of this mission. The Declaration of Geneva of the World Medical Association binds the physician with the words, "The health of my patient will be my first consideration," and the International Code of Medical Ethics declares that, "A physician shall act only in the patient's interest when providing medical care which might have the effect of weakening the physical and mental condition of the patient."

The purpose of biomedical research involving human subjects must be to improve diagnostic, therapeutic and prophylactic procedures and the understanding of the aetiology and pathogenesis of disease.

In current medical practice most diagnostic, therapeutic or prophylactic procedures involve hazards. This applies especially to biomedical research. Medical progress is based on research which ultimately must rest in part on experimentation involving human subjects.

In the field of biomedical research a fundamental distinction must be recognized between medical research in which the aim is essentially diagnostic or therapeutic for a patient, and medical research, the essential object of which is purely scientific and without implying direct diagnostic or therapeutic value to the person subjected to the research.

Special caution must be exercised in the conduct of research which may affect the environment, and the welfare of animals used for research must be respected.

Because it is essential that the results of laboratory experiments be applied to human beings to further scientific knowledge and to help suffering humanity, the World Medical Association has prepared the following recommendations as a guide to every physician in

157

biomedical research involving human subjects. They should be kept under review in the future. It must be stressed that the standards as drafted are only a guide to physicians all over the world. Physicians are not relieved from criminal, civil and ethical responsibilities under the laws of their own countries.

I. Basic Principles

1. Biomedical research involving human subjects must conform to generally accepted scientific principles and should be based on adequately performed laboratory and animal experimentation and on a thorough knowledge of the scientific literature.

2. The design and performance of each experimental procedure involving human subjects should be clearly formulated in an experimental protocol which should be transmitted for consideration, comment and guidance to a specially appointed committee independent of the investigator and the sponsor provided that this independent committee is in conformity with the laws and regulations of the country in which the research experiment is performed.

3. Biomedical research involving human subjects should be conducted only by scientifically qualified persons and under the supervision of a clinically competent medical person. The responsibility for the human subject must always rest with a medically qualified person and never rest on the subject of the research, even though the subject has given his or her consent.

4. Biomedical research involving human subjects cannot legitimately be carried out unless the importance of the objective is in proportion to the inherent risk to the subject.

5. Every biomedical research project involving human subjects should be preceded by careful assessment of predictable risks in comparison with foreseeable benefits to the subject or to others. Concern for the interests of the subject must always prevail over the interests of science and society.

6. The right of the research subject to safeguard his or her integrity must always be respected. Every precaution should be taken to respect the privacy of the subject and to minimize the impact of the study on the subject's physical and mental integrity and on the personality of the subject.

7. Physicians should abstain from engaging in research projects involving human subjects unless they are satisfied that the hazards involved are believed to be predictable. Physicians should cease any investigation if the hazards are found to outweigh the potential benefits.

8. In publication of the results of his or her research, the physician is obliged to preserve the accuracy of the results. Reports of experimentation not in accordance with the principles laid down in this Declaration should not be accepted for publication.

9. In any research on human beings, each potential subject must be adequately informed of the aims, methods, anticipated benefits and potential hazards of the study and the discomfort it may entail. He or she should be informed that he or she is at liberty to abstain from participation in the study and that he or she is free to withdraw his or her consent to participation at any time. The physician should then obtain the subject's freely-given informed consent, preferably in writing.

10. When obtaining informed consent for the research project the physician should be particularly cautious if the subject is in a dependent relationship to him or her or may consent under duress. In that case the informed consent should be obtained by a physician who is not engaged in the investigation and who is completely independent of this official relationship.

11. In case of legal incompetence, informed consent should be obtained from the legal guardian in accordance with national legislation. Where physical or mental incapacity makes it impossible to obtain informed consent, or when the subject is a minor, permission from the responsible relative replaces that of the subject in accordance with national legislation.Whenever the minor child is in fact able to give a consent, the minor's consent must be obtained in addition to the consent of the minor's legal guardian.

12. The research protocol should always contain a statement of the ethical considerations involved and should indicate that the principles enunciated in the present Declaration

are complied with.

II. Medical Research Combined with Professional Care (Clinical Research)

1. In the treatment of the sick person, the physician must be free to use a new diagnostic and therapeutic measure, if in his or her judgment it offers hope of saving life, reestablishing health or alleviating suffering.

2. The potential benefits, hazards and discomfort of a new method should be weighed against the advantages of the best current diagnostic and therapeutic methods.

3. In any medical study, every patient—including those of a control group, if any—should be assured of the best proven diagnostic and therapeutic method.

4. The refusal of the patient to participate in a study must never interfere with the physician-patient relationship.

5. If the physician considers it essential not to obtain informed consent, the specific reasons for this proposal should be stated in the experimental protocol for transmission to the independent committee (I, 2).

6. The physician can combine medical research with professional care, the objective being the acquisition of new medical knowledge, only to the extent that medical research is justified by its potential diagnostic or therapeutic value for the patient.

III. Non-Therapeutic Biomedical Research Involving Human Subjects (Non-Clinical Biomedical Research)

1. In the purely scientific application of medical research carried out on a human being, it is the duty of the physician to remain the protector of the life and health of that person on whom biomedical research is being carried out.

2. The subjects should be volunteers—either healthy persons or patients for whom the experimental design is not related to the patient's illness.

3. The investigator or the investigating team should discontinue the research if in his/her or their judgment it may, if continued, be harmful to the individual.

4. In research on man, the interest of science and society should never take precedence over considerations related to the well-being of the subject.

(Collection of information requirements approved by the Office of Management and Budget under control number 0910-0014)

[52 FR 8831, Mar. 19, 1987, as amended at 52 FR 23031, June 17, 1987; 56 FR 22113, May 14, 1991]

Sec. 312.130 Availability for public disclosure of data and information in an IND.

(a) The existence of an investigational new drug application will not be disclosed by FDA unless it has previously been publicly disclosed or acknowledged.

(b) The availability for public disclosure of all data and information in an investigational new drug application for a new drug or antibiotic drug will be handled in accordance with the provisions established in Sec. 314.430 for the confidentiality of data and information in applications submitted in part 314. The availability for public disclosure of all data and information in an investigational new drug application for a biological product will be governed by the provisions of Secs. 601.50 and 601.51.

(c) Notwithstanding the provisions of Sec. 314.430, FDA shall disclose upon request to an individual to whom an investigational new drug has been given a copy of any IND safety report relating to the use in the individual.

(d) The availability of information required to be publicly disclosed for investigations involving an exception from informed consent under Sec. 50.24 of this chapter will be handled as follows: Persons wishing to request the publicly disclosable information in the IND that was required to be filed in Docket Number 95S-0158 in the Dockets Management Branch (HFA-305), Food and Drug Administration, 12420 Parklawn Dr., rm. 1-23, Rockville, MD 20857, shall submit a request under the Freedom of Information Act.

[52 FR 8831, Mar. 19, 1987. Redesignated at 53 FR 41523, Oct. 21, 1988, as amended at 61 FR 51530, Oct. 2, 1996]

Sec. 312.140 Address for correspondence.

(a) Except as provided in paragraph (b) of this section, a sponsor shall send an initial IND submission to the Central Document Room, Center for Drug Evaluation and Research, Food and Drug Administration, Park Bldg., Rm. 214, 12420 Parklawn Dr., Rockville, MD 20852. On receiving the IND, FDA will inform the sponsor which one of the divisions in the Center' for Drug Evaluation and Research or the Center for Biologics Evaluation and Research is responsible for the IND. Amendments, reports, and other correspondence relating to matters covered by the IND should be directed to the appropriate division. The outside wrapper of each submission shall state what is contained in the submission, for example, "IND Application", "Protocol Amendment", etc.

(b) Applications for the products listed below should be submitted to the Division of Biological Investigational New Drugs (HFB-230), Center for Biologics Evaluation and Research, Food and Drug Administration, 8800 Rockville Pike, Bethesda, MD 20892. (1) Products subject to the licensing provisions of the Public Health Service Act of July 1, 1944 (58 Stat. 682, as amended (42 U.S.C. 201 et seq.)) or subject to part 600; (2) ingredients packaged together with containers intended for the collection, processing, or storage of blood or blood components; (3) urokinase products; (4) plasma volume expanders and hydroxyethyl starch for leukapheresis; and (5) coupled antibodies, i.e., products that consist of an antibody component coupled with a drug or radionuclide component in which both components provide a pharmacological effect but the biological component determines the site of action.

(c) All correspondence relating to biological products for human use which are also radioactive drugs shall be submitted to the Division of Oncology and Radiopharmaceutical Drug Products (HFD-150), Center for Drug Evaluation and Research, Food and Drug Administration, 5600 Fishers Lane, Rockville, MD 20857, except that applications for coupled antibodies shall be submitted in accordance with paragraph (b) of this section.

(d) All correspondence relating to export of an investigational drug under Sec. 312.110(b)(2) shall be submitted to the International Affairs Staff (HFY-50), Office of Health Affairs, Food and Drug Administration, 5600 Fishers Lane, Rockville, MD 20857.

(Collection of information requirements approved by the Office of Management and Budget under control number 0910-0014)

[52 FR 8831, Mar. 19, 1987, as amended at 52 FR 23031, June 17, 1987; 55 FR 11580, Mar. 29, 1990]

Sec. 312.145 Guidelines.

(a) FDA has made available guidelines under Sec. 10.90(b) to help persons to comply with certain requirements of this part.

(b) The Center for Drug Evaluation and Research and the Center for Biologics Evaluation and Research maintain lists of guidelines that apply to the Centers' regulations. The lists state how a person can obtain a copy of each guideline. A request for a copy of the lists should be directed to the CDER Executive Secretariat Staff (HFD-8), Center for Drug Evaluation and Research, Food and Drug Administration, 5600 Fishers Lane, Rockville, MD 20857, for drug products, and the Congressional, Consumer, and International Affairs Staff (HFB-142), Center for Biologics Evaluation and Research, Food and Drug Administration, 8800 Rockville Pike, Bethesda, MD 20892, for biological products.

[52 FR 8831, Mar. 19, 1987, as amended at 55 FR 11580, Mar. 29, 1990; 56 FR 3776, Jan. 31, 1991; 57 FR 10814, Mar. 31, 1992]

Subpart G—Drugs for Investigational Use in Laboratory Research Animals or In Vitro Tests

Sec. 312.160 Drugs for investigational use in laboratory research animals or in vitro tests.

(a) Authorization to ship. (1)(i) A person may ship a drug intended solely for tests in vitro or in animals used only for laboratory research purposes if it is labeled as follows:

CAUTION: Contains a new drug for investigational use only in laboratory research animals, or for tests in vitro. Not for use in humans.

(ii) A person may ship a biological product for investigational in vitro diagnostic use that is listed in Sec. 312.2(b)(2)(ii) if it is labeled as follows:

CAUTION: Contains a biological product for investigational in vitro diagnostic tests only.

(2) A person shipping a drug under paragraph (a) of this section shall use due diligence to assure that the consignee is regularly engaged in conducting such tests and that the shipment of the new drug will actually be used for tests in vitro or in animals used only for laboratory research.

(3) A person who ships a drug under paragraph (a) of this section shall maintain adequate records showing the name and post office address of the expert to whom the drug is shipped and the date, quantity, and batch or code mark of each shipment and delivery. Records of shipments under paragraph (a)(1)(i) of this section are to be maintained for a period of 2 years after the shipment. Records and reports of data and shipments under paragraph (a)(1)(ii) of this section are to be maintained in accordance with Sec. 312.57(b). The person who ships the drug shall upon request from any properly authorized officer or employee of the Food and Drug Administration, at reasonable times, permit such officer or employee to have access to and copy and verify records required to be maintained under this section.

(b) Termination of authorization to ship. FDA may terminate authorization to ship a drug under this section if it finds that:

(1) The sponsor of the investigation has failed to comply with any of the conditions for shipment established under this section; or

(2) The continuance of the investigation is unsafe or otherwise contrary to the public interest or the drug is used for purposes other than bona fide scientific investigation. FDA will notify the person shipping the drug of its finding and invite immediate correction. If correction is not immediately made, the person shall have an opportunity for a regulatory hearing before FDA pursuant to part 16.

(c) Disposition of unused drug. The person who ships the drug under paragraph (a) of this section shall assure the return of all unused supplies of the drug from individual investigators whenever the investigation discontinues or the investigation is terminated. The person who ships the drug may authorize in writing alternative disposition of unused supplies of the drug provided this alternative disposition does not expose humans to risks from the drug, either directly or indirectly (e.g., through food-producing animals). The shipper shall maintain records of any alternative disposition.

(Collection of information requirements approved by the Office of Management and Budget under control number 0910-0014)

[52 FR 8831, Mar. 19, 1987, as amended at 52 FR 23031, June 17, 1987. Redesignated at 53 FR 41523, Oct. 21, 1988]

PART 600—BIOLOGICAL PRODUCTS

Subpart A—General Provisions

Sec. 600.3 Definitions.

As used in this subchapter:

(a) *Act* means the Public Health Service Act (58 Stat. 682), approved July 1, 1944.

(b) *Secretary* means the Secretary of Health and Human Services and any other officer or employee of the Department of Health and Human Services to whom the authority involved has been delegated.

(c) *Commissioner of Food and Drugs* means the Commissioner of the Food and Drug Administration.

(d) *Center for Biologics Evaluation and Research* means Center for Biologics Evaluation and Research of the Food and Drug Administration.

(e) *State* means a State or the District of Columbia, Puerto Rico, or the Virgin Islands.

(f) *Possession* includes among other possessions, Puerto Rico and the Virgin Islands.

(g) *Products* includes biological products and trivalent organic arsenicals.

(h) *Biological product* means any virus, therapeutic serum, toxin, antitoxin, or analogous product applicable to the prevention, treatment or cure of diseases or injuries of man:

(1) A *virus* is interpreted to be a product containing the minute living cause of an infectious disease and includes but is not limited to filterable viruses, bacteria, rickettsia, fungi, and protozoa.

(2) A *therapeutic serum* is a product obtained from blood by removing the clot or clot components and the blood cells.

(3) A *toxin* is a product containing a soluble substance poisonous to laboratory animals or to man in doses of 1 milliliter or less (or equivalent in weight) of the product, and having the property, following the injection of non-fatal doses into an animal, of causing to be produced therein another soluble substance which specifically neutralizes the poisonous substance and which is demonstrable in the serum of the animal thus immunized.

(4) An *antitoxin* is a product containing the soluble substance in serum or other body fluid of an immunized animal which specifically neutralizes the toxin against which the animal is immune.

(5) A product is *analogous*:

(i) To a *virus* if prepared from or with a virus or agent actually or potentially infectious, without regard to the degree of virulence or toxicogenicity of the specific strain used.

(ii) To a *therapeutic serum*, if composed of whole blood or plasma or containing some organic constituent or product other than a hormone or an amino acid, derived from whole blood, plasma, or serum.

(iii) To a *toxin or antitoxin*, if intended, irrespective of its source of origin, to be applicable to the prevention, treatment, or cure of disease or injuries of man through a specific immune process.

(i) *Trivalent organic arsenicals* means arsphenamine and its derivatives (or any other trivalent organic arsenic compound) applicable to the prevention, treatment, or cure of diseases or injuries of man.

(j) A product is deemed applicable to the prevention, treatment, or cure of diseases or injuries of man irrespective of the mode of administration or application recommended, including use when intended through administration or application to a person as an aid in diagnosis, or in evaluating the degree of susceptibility or immunity possessed by a person, and including also any other use for purposes of diagnosis if the diagnostic substance so used is prepared from or with the aid of a biological product.

(k) *Proper name*, as applied to a product, means the name designated in the license for use upon each package of the product.

(l) Dating period means the period beyond which the product cannot be expected beyond reasonable doubt to yield its specific results.

(m) Expiration date means the calendar month and year, and where applicable, the day and hour, that the dating period ends.

(n) The word standards means specifications and procedures applicable to an establishment or to the manufacture or release of products, which are prescribed in this subchapter and which are designed to insure the continued safety, purity and potency of such products.

(o) The word continued as applied to the safety, purity and potency of products is interpreted to apply to the dating period.

(p) The word safety means the relative freedom from harmful effect to persons affected, directly or indirectly, by a product when prudently administered, taking into consideration the character of the product in relation to the condition of the recipient at the time.

(q) The word sterility is interpreted to mean freedom from viable contaminating microorganisms, as determined by the tests prescribed in Sec. 610.12 of this chapter.

(r) Purity means relative freedom from extraneous matter in the finished product, whether or not harmful to the recipient or deleterious to the product. Purity includes but is not limited to relative freedom from residual moisture or other volatile substances and pyrogenic substances.

(s) The word potency is interpreted to mean the specific ability or capacity of the product, as indicated by appropriate laboratory tests or by adequately controlled clinical data obtained through the administration of the product in the manner intended, to effect a given result.

(t) Manufacturer means any legal person or entity engaged in the manufacture of a product subject to license under the act; "Manufacturer" also includes any legal person or entity who is an applicant for a license where the applicant assumes responsibility for compliance with the applicable product and establishment standards.

(u) Manufacture means all steps in propagation or manufacture and preparation of products and includes but is not limited to filling, testing, labeling, packaging, and storage by the manufacturer.

(v) Location includes all buildings, appurtenances, equipment and animals used, and personnel engaged by a manufacturer within a particular area designated by an address adequate for identification.

(w) Establishment includes all locations.

(x) Lot means that quantity of uniform material identified by the manufacturer as having been thoroughly mixed in a single vessel.

(y) A filling refers to a group of final containers identical in all respects, which have been filled with the same product from the same bulk lot without any change that will affect the integrity of the filling assembly.

(z) Process refers to a manufacturing step that is performed on the product itself which may affect its safety, purity or potency, in contrast to such manufacturing steps which do not affect intrinsically the safety, purity or potency of the product.

(aa) Selling agent or distributor means any person engaged in the unrestricted distribution, other than by sale at retail, of products subject to license.

(bb) Container (referred to also as "final container") is the immediate unit, bottle, vial, ampule, tube, or other receptacle containing the product as distributed for sale, barter, or exchange.

(cc) Package means the immediate carton, receptacle, or wrapper, including all labeling matter therein and thereon, and the contents of the one or more enclosed containers. If no package, as defined in the preceding sentence, is used, the container shall be deemed to be the package.

(dd) Label means any written, printed, or graphic matter on the container or package or any such matter clearly visible through the immediate carton, receptacle, or wrapper.

(ee) Radioactive biological product means a biological product which is labeled with a radionuclide or intended solely to be labeled with a radionuclide.

(ff) Amendment is the submission of information to a pending license application or supplement, to revise or modify the application as originally submitted.

(gg) Supplement is a request to the Director, Center for Biologics Evaluation and Research, to approve a change in an approved license application.

[38 FR 32048, Nov. 20, 1973, as amended at 40 FR 31313, July 25, 1975; 55 FR 11014, Mar. 26, 1990; 61 FR 24232, May 14, 1996; 62 FR 39901, July 24, 1997]

Subpart B—Establishment Standards

Sec. 600.10 Personnel.

(a) [Reserved]

(b) Personnel. Personnel shall have capabilities commensurate with their assigned functions, a thorough understanding of the manufacturing operations which they perform, the necessary training and experience relating to individual products, and adequate information concerning the application of the pertinent provisions of this subchapter to the irrespective functions. Personnel shall include such professionally trained persons as are necessary to insure the competent performance of all manufacturing processes.

(c) Restrictions on personnel—(1) Specific duties. Persons who sepresence can affect adversely the safety and purity of a product shall be excluded from the room where the manufacture of a product is in progress.

(2) Sterile operations. Personnel performing sterile operations shall wear clean or sterilized protective clothing and devices to the extent necessary to protect the product from contamination.

(3) Pathogenic viruses and spore-bearing organisms. Persons working with viruses pathogenic for man or with spore-bearing microorganisms, and persons engaged in the care of animals or animal quarters, shall be excluded from areas where other products are manufactured, or such persons shall change outer clothing, including shoes, or wear protective covering prior to entering such areas.

(4) Live vaccine work areas. Persons may not enter a live vaccine processing area after having worked with other infectious agents in any other laboratory during the same working day. Only persons actually concerned with propagation of the culture, production of the vaccine, and unit maintenance, shall be allowed in live vaccine processing areas when active work is in progress. Casual visitors shall be excluded from such units at all times and all others having business in such areas shall be admitted only under supervision. Street clothing, including shoes, shall be replaced or covered by suitable laboratory clothing before entering a live vaccine processing unit. Persons caring for animals used in the manufacture of live vaccines shall be excluded from other animal quarters and from contact with other animals during the same working day.

[38 FR 32048, Nov. 20, 1973, as amended at 49 FR 23833, June 8, 1984; 55 FR 11014, Mar. 26, 1990; 62 FR 53538, Oct. 15, 1997]

Sec. 600.11 Physical establishment, equipment, animals, and care.

(a) Work areas. All rooms and work areas where products are manufactured or stored shall be kept orderly, clean, and free of dirt, dust, vermin and objects not required for manufacturing. Precautions shall be taken to avoid clogging and back-siphonage of drainage systems. Precautions shall be taken to exclude extraneous infectious agents from manufacturing areas. Work rooms shall be well lighted and ventilated. The ventilation system shall be arranged so as to prevent the dissemination of microorganisms from one manufacturing area to another and to avoid other conditions unfavorable to the safety of the product. Filling rooms, and other rooms where open, sterile operations are conducted, shall be adequate to meet manufacturing needs and such rooms shall be constructed and equipped to permit thorough cleaning and to keep air-borne contaminants at a minimum. If such rooms are used for other purposes, they shall be cleaned and prepared prior to use for sterile operations. Refrigerators, incubators and warm rooms shall be maintained at temperatures within applicable ranges and shall be free of extraneous material which might affect the safety of the product.

(b) Equipment. Apparatus for sterilizing equipment and the method of operation shall be such as to insure the destruction of contaminating microorganisms. The effectiveness of the sterilization procedure shall be no less than that achieved by an attained temperature of 121.5 deg. C maintained for 20 minutes by saturated steam or by an attained temperature of 170 deg. C maintained for 2 hours with dry heat. Processing and storage containers, filters, filling apparatus, and other pieces of apparatus and accessory equipment, including pipes and tubing, shall be designed and constructed to permit thorough cleaning and, where possible, inspection for cleanliness. All surfaces that come in contact with products shall be clean and free of surface solids, leachable contaminants, and other materials that will hasten the deterioration of the product or otherwise render it less suitable for the intended use. For products for which sterility is a factor, equipment shall be sterile, unless sterility of the product is assured by subsequent procedures.

(c) Laboratory and bleeding rooms. Rooms used for the processing of products, including bleeding rooms, shall be effectively fly-proofed and kept free of flies and vermin. Such rooms shall be so constructed as to insure freedom from dust, smoke and other deleterious substances and to permit thorough cleaning and disinfection. Rooms for animal injection and bleeding, and rooms for smallpox vaccine animals, shall be disinfected and be provided with the necessary water, electrical and other services.

(d) Animal quarters and stables. Animal quarters, stables and food storage areas shall be of appropriate construction, fly-proofed, adequately lighted and ventilated, and maintained in a clean, vermin-free and sanitary condition. No manure or refuse shall be stored as to permit the breeding of flies on the premises, nor shall the establishment be located in close proximity to off-property manure or refuse storage capable of engendering fly breeding.

(e) Restrictions on building and equipment use—(1) Work of a diagnostic nature. Laboratory procedures of a clinical diagnostic nature involving materials that may be contaminated, shall not be performed in space used for the manufacture of products except that manufacturing space which is used only occasionally may be used for diagnostic work provided spore-bearing pathogenic microorganisms are not involved and provided the space is thoroughly cleaned and disinfected before the manufacture of products is resumed.

(2) Spore-bearing organisms for supplemental sterilization procedure control test. Spore-bearing organisms used as an additional control in sterilization procedures may be introduced into areas used for the manufacture of products, only for the purposes of the test and only immediately before use for such purposes: Provided, That (i) the organism is not pathogenic for man or animals and does not produce pyrogens or toxins, (ii) the culture is demonstrated to be pure, (iii) transfer of test cultures to culture media shall be limited to the sterility test area or areas designated for work with spore-bearing organisms, (iv) each culture be labeled with the name of the microorganism and the statement "Caution: microbial spores. See directions for storage, use and disposition.", and (v) the container of each culture is designed to withstand handling without breaking.

(3) Work with spore-bearing organisms. Except as provided in the previous paragraph, all work with spore-bearing microorganisms shall be done in an entirely separate building: Provided, That such work may be done in a portion of a building used in the manufacture of products not containing spore-bearing microorganisms if such portion is completely walled-off and is constructed so as to prevent contamination of other areas and if entrances to such portion are independent of the remainder of the building. All vessels, apparatus and equipment used for spore-bearing microorganisms shall be permanently identified and reserved exclusively for use with those organisms. Materials destined for further manufacturing may be removed from such an area only under conditions which will prevent the introduction of spores into other manufacturing areas.

(4) Live vaccine processing. Space used for processing a live vaccine shall not be used for any other purpose during the processing period for that vaccine and such space shall be

decontaminated prior to initiation of the processing. Live vaccine processing areas shall be isolated from and independent of any space used for any other purpose by being either in a separate building, in a separate wing of a building, or in quarters at the blind end of a corridor and shall include adequate space and equipment for all processing steps up to filling into final containers. Test procedures which potentially involve the presence of microorganisms other than the vaccine strains, or the use of tissue culture cell lines other than primary cultures, shall not be conducted in space used for processing live vaccine.

(5) Equipment and supplies—contamination. Equipment and supplies used in work on or otherwise exposed to any pathogenic or potentially pathogenic agent shall be kept separated from equipment and supplies used in the manufacture of products to the extent necessary to prevent cross-contamination.

(f) Animals used in manufacture—(1) Care of animals used in manufacturing. Caretakers and attendants for animals used for the manufacture of products shall be sufficient in number and have adequate experience to insure adequate care. Animal quarters and cages shall be kept in sanitary condition. Animals on production shall be inspected daily to observe response to production procedures. Animals that become ill for reasons not related to production shall be isolated from other animals and shall not be used for production until recovery is complete. Competent veterinary care shall be provided as needed.

(2) Quarantine of animals—(i) General. No animal shall be used in processing unless kept under competent daily inspection and preliminary quarantine for a period of at least 7 days before use, or as otherwise provided in this subchapter. Only healthy animals free from detectable communicable diseases shall be used. Animals must remain in overt good health throughout the quarantine periods and particular care shall be taken during the quarantine periods to reject animals of the equine genus which may be infected with glanders and animals which may be infected with tuberculosis.

(ii) Quarantine of monkeys. In addition to observing the pertinent general quarantine requirements, monkeys used as a source of tissue in the manufacture of vaccine shall be maintained in quarantine for at least 6 weeks prior to use, except when otherwise provided in this part. Only monkeys that have reacted negatively to tuberculin at the start of the quarantine period and again within 2 weeks prior to use shall be used in the manufacture of vaccine. Due precaution shall be taken to prevent cross-infection from any infected or potentially infected monkeys on the premises. Monkeys to be used in the manufacture of a live vaccine shall be maintained throughout the quarantine period in cages closed on all sides with solid materials except the front which shall be screened, with no more than two monkeys housed in one cage. Cage mates shall not be interchanged.

(3) Immunization against tetanus. Horses and other animals susceptible to tetanus, that are used in the processing steps of the manufacture of biological products, shall be treated adequately to maintain immunity to tetanus.

(4) Immunization and bleeding of animals used as a source of products. Toxins or other nonviable antigens administered in the immunization of animals used in the manufacture of products shall be sterile. Viable antigens, when so used, shall be free of contaminants, as determined by appropriate tests prior to use. Injections shall not be made into horses within 6 inches of bleeding site. Horses shall not be bled for manufacturing purposes while showing persistent general reaction or local reaction near the site of bleeding. Blood shall not be used if it was drawn within 5 days of injecting the animals with viable microorganisms. Animals shall not be bled for manufacturing purposes when they have an intercurrent disease. Blood intended for use as a source of a biological product shall be collected in clean, sterile vessels. When the product is intended for use by injection, such vessels shall also be pyrogen-free.

(5) [Reserved]

(6) Reporting of certain diseases. In cases of actual or suspected infection with foot and mouth disease, glanders, tetanus, anthrax, gas gangrene, equine infectious anemia; equine encephalomyelitis, or any of the pock diseases among animals intended for use or used in the manufacture of products, the manufacturer shall immediately notify the Director, Center for Biologics Evaluation and Research.

(7) Monkeys used previously for experimental or test purposes. Monkeys that have been used previously for experimental or test purposes with live microbiological agents shall not be used as a source of kidney tissue for the manufacture of vaccine. Except as provided otherwise in this subchapter, monkeys that have been used previously for other experimental or test purposes may be used as a source of kidney tissue upon their return to a normal condition, provided all quarantine requirements have been met.

(8) Necropsy examination of monkeys. Each monkey used in the manufacture of vaccine shall be examined at necropsy under the direction of a qualified pathologist, physician, or veterinarian having experience with diseases of monkeys, for evidence of ill health, particularly for (i) evidence of tuberculosis, (ii) presence of herpes-like lesions, including eruptions or plaques on or around the lips, in the buccal cavity or on the gums, and (iii) signs of conjunctivitis. If there are any such signs or other significant gross pathological lesions, the tissue shall not be used in the manufacture of vaccine.

(g) Filling procedures. Filling procedures shall be such as will not affect adversely the safety, purity or potency of the product.

(h) Containers and closures. All final containers and closures shall be made of material that will not hasten the deterioration of the product or otherwise render it less suitable for the intended use. All final containers and closures shall be clean and free of surface solids, leachable contaminants and other materials that will hasten the deterioration of the product or otherwise render it less suitable for the intended use. After filling, sealing shall be performed in a manner that will maintain the integrity of the product during the dating period. In addition, final containers and closures for products intended for use by injection shall be sterile and free from pyrogens. Except as otherwise provided in the regulations of this subchapter, final containers for products intended for use by injection shall be colorless and sufficiently transparent to permit visual examination of the contents under normal light. As soon as possible after filling final containers shall be labeled as prescribed in Sec. 610.60 et seq. of this chapter, except that final containers may be stored without such prescribed labeling provided they are stored in a sealed receptacle labeled both inside and outside with at least the name of the product, the lot number, and the filling identification.

[38 FR 32048, Nov. 20, 1973, as amended at 41 FR 10428, Mar. 11, 1976; 49 FR 23833, June 8, 1984; 55 FR 11013, Mar. 26, 1990]

Sec. 600.12 Records.

(a) Maintenance of records. Records shall be made, concurrently with the performance, of each step in the manufacture and distribution of products, in such a manner that at any time successive steps in the manufacture and distribution of any lot may be traced by an inspector. Such records shall be legible and indelible, shall identify the person immediately responsible, shall include dates of the various steps, and be as detailed as necessary for clear understanding of each step by one experienced in the manufacture of products.

(b) Records retention—(1) General. Records shall be retained for such interval beyond the expiration date as is necessary for the individual product, to permit the return of any clinical report of unfavorable reactions. The retention period shall be no less than five years after the records of manufacture have been completed or six months after the latest expiration date for the individual product, whichever represents a later date.

(2) Records of recall. Complete records shall be maintained pertaining to the recall from distribution of any product upon notification by the Director, Center for Biologics Evaluation and Research, to recall for failure to conform with the standards prescribed in the regulations of this subchapter, because of deterioration of the product or for any other factor by reason of which the distribution of the product would constitute a danger to health.

(3) Suspension of requirement for retention. The Director, Center for Biologics Evaluation and Research, may authorize the suspension of the requirement to retain records of a specific manufacturing step upon a showing that such records no longer have significance for the purposes for which they were made: Provided, That a summary of such records shall be retained.

(c) Records of sterilization of equipment and supplies. Records relating to the mode of sterilization, date, duration, temperature and other conditions relating to each sterilization of equipment and supplies used in the processing of products shall be made by means of automatic recording devices or by means of a system of recording which gives equivalent assurance of the accuracy and reliability of the record. Such records shall be maintained in a manner that permits an identification of the product with the particular manufacturing process to which the sterilization relates.

(d) Animal necropsy records. A necropsy record shall be kept on each animal from which a biological product has been obtained and which dies or is sacrificed while being so used.

(e) Records in case of divided manufacturing responsibility. If two or more establishments participate in the manufacture of a product, the records of each such establishment must show plainly the degree of its responsibility. In addition, each participating manufacturer shall furnish to the manufacturer who prepares the product in final form for sale, barter or exchange, a copy of all records relating to the manufacturing operations performed by such participating manufacturer insofar as they concern the safety, purity and potency of the lots of the product involved, and the manufacturer who prepares the product in final form shall retain a complete record of all the manufacturing operations relating to the product.

[38 FR 32048, Nov. 20, 1973, as amended at 49 FR 23833, June 8, 1984; 55 FR 11013, Mar. 26, 1990]

Sec. 600.13 Retention samples.

Manufacturers shall retain for a period of at least 6 months after the expiration date, unless a different time period is specified in additional standards, a quantity of representative material of each lot of each product, sufficient for examination and testing for safety and potency, except Whole Blood, Cryoprecipitated AHF, Platelets, Red Blood Cells, Plasma, and Source Plasma and Allergenic Products prepared to a physician's prescription. Samples so retained shall be selected at random from either final container material, or from bulk and final containers, provided they include at least one final container as a final package, or package-equivalent of such filling of each lot of the product as intended for distribution. Such sample material shall be stored at temperatures and under conditions which will maintain the identity and integrity of the product. Samples retained as required in this section shall be in addition to samples of specific products required to be submitted to the Center for Biologics Evaluation and Research. Exceptions may be authorized by the Director, Center for Biologics Evaluation and Research, when the lot yields relatively few final containers and when such lots are prepared by the same method in large number and in close succession.

Sec. 600.14 Reporting of errors.

(a) The Director, Office of Compliance, Center for Biologics Evaluation and Research (HFB-100), 8800 Rockville Pike, Bethesda, MD 20892, shall be notified promptly of errors or accidents in the manufacture of products that may affect the safety, purity, or potency of any product.

(b) Manufacturers of licensed in vitro diagnostic products, and manufacturers of unlicensed in vitro diagnostic products which are required to be registered under part 607 of this chapter, shall notify the Director in accordance with paragraph (a) of this section. Manufacturers of other in vitro diagnostic products which are required to be registered under part 807 of this chapter, shall report in accordance with part 803 of this chapter.

[38 FR 32048, Nov. 20, 1973, as amended at 49 FR 23833, June 8, 1984; 49 FR 36348, Sept. 14, 1984; 55 FR 11014, Mar. 26, 1990]

Sec. 600.15 Temperatures during shipment.

The following products shall be maintained during shipment at the specified temperatures:

(a) Products.

Product	Temperature
Cryoprecipitated AHF	-18 °C or colder.
Measles and Rubella Virus Vaccine Live	10 °C or colder.
Measles Live and Smallpox Vaccine	Do.
Measles, Mumps, and Rubella Virus Vaccine Live	Do.
Measles and Mumps Virus Vaccine Live	Do.
Measles Virus Vaccine Live	Do.
Mumps Virus Vaccine Live	Do.
Fresh Frozen Plasma	-18 °C or colder.
Liquid Plasma	1 to 10 °C.
Plasma	-18 °C or colder.
Platelet Rich Plasma	Between 1 and 10 °C if the label indicates storage label indicates storage between 1 and 6 °C, or all reasonable methods to maintain the temperature as close as possible to a range between 20 and 24 °C, if the label indicates storage between 20 and 24 °C.
Platelets	Between 1 and 10 °C if the label indicates storage between 1 and 6 °C, or all reasonable methods to maintain the temperature as close as possible to a range between 20 to 24 °C, if the label indicates storage between 20 and 24 °C.
Poliovirus Vaccine Live Oral Trivalent	0 °C or colder.
Poliovirus Vaccine Live Oral Type I	Do.
Poliovirus Vaccine Live Oral Type II	Do.
Poliovirus Vaccine Live Oral Type III	Do.
Red Blood Cells (liquid product)	Between 1 and 10 °C.
Red Blood Cells Frozen	-65 °C or colder.
Rubella and Mumps Virus Vaccine Live	10 °C or colder.
Rubella Virus Vaccine Live	Do.
Smallpox Vaccine (Liquid Product)	0 °C or colder.
Source Plasma	-5 °C or colder.
Source Plasma Liquid	10 °C or colder.
Whole Blood	Blood that is transported from the collecting facility to the processing facility shall be transported in an environment capable of continuously cooling the blood toward a temperature range of 1 to 10 °C, or at a temperature as close as possible to 20 to 24 °C for a period not to exceed 6 hours. Blood transported from the storage facility shall be placed in an appropriate environment to maintain a temperature range between 1 to 10 °C during shipment.
Yellow Fever Vaccine	0 C or colder.

(b) Exemptions. Exemptions or modifications shall be made only upon written approval, in the form of a supplement of the product license, issued by the Director, Center for Biologics Evaluation and Research.

[39 FR 39872, Nov. 12, 1974, as amended at 49 FR 23833, June 8, 1984; 50 FR 4133, Jan. 29, 1985; 50 FR 9000, Mar. 6, 1985; 55 FR 11013, Mar. 26, 1990; 59 FR 49351, Sept. 28, 1994]

Subpart C—Establishment Inspection

Sec. 600.20 Inspectors.

Inspections shall be made by an officer of the Food and Drug Administration having special knowledge of the methods used in the manufacture and control of products and designated for such purposes by the Commissioner of Food and Drugs, or by any officer, agent, or employee of the Department of Health and Human Services specifically designated for such purpose by the Secretary.

[38 FR 32048, Nov. 20, 1973]

Sec. 600.21 Time of inspection.

The inspection of an establishment for which a license is pending need not be made until the establishment is in operation and is manufacturing the complete product for which a product license is desired. In case the license is denied following inspection for the original license, no reinspection need be made until assurance has been received that the faulty conditions which were the basis of the denial have been corrected. An inspection of each licensed establishment and its additional location(s) shall be made at least once every 2 years. Inspections may be made with or without notice, and shall be made during regular business hours unless otherwise directed.

[38 FR 32048, Nov. 20, 1973, as amended at 48 FR 26314, June 7, 1983]

Sec. 600.22 Duties of inspector.

The inspector shall:

(a) Call upon the active head of the establishment, stating the object of his visit,

(b) Interrogate the proprietor or other personnel of the establishment as he may deem necessary,

(c) Examine the details of location, construction, equipment and maintenance, including stables, barns, warehouses, manufacturing laboratories, bleeding clinics maintained for the collection of human blood, shipping rooms, record rooms, and any other structure or appliance used in any part of the manufacture of a product,

(d) Investigate as fully as he deems necessary the methods of propagation, processing, testing, storing, dispensing, recording, or other details of manufacture and distribution of each licensed product, or product for which a license has been requested, including observation of these procedures in actual operation,

(e) Obtain and cause to be sent to the Director, Center for Biologics Evaluation and Research, adequate samples for the examination of any product or ingredient used in its manufacture,

(f) Bring to the attention of the manufacturer any fault observed in the course of inspection in location, construction, manufacturing methods, or administration of a licensed establishment which might lead to impairment of a product,

(g) Inspect and copy, as circumstances may require, any records required to be kept pursuant to Sec. 600.12,

(h) Certify as to the condition of the establishment and of the manufacturing methods followed and make recommendations as to action deemed appropriate with respect to any application for license or any license previously issued.

[38 FR 32048, Nov. 20, 1973, as amended at 49 FR 23833, June 8, 1984; 55 FR 11013, Mar. 26, 1990]

Subpart D—Reporting of Adverse Experiences

Sec. 600.80 Postmarketing reporting of adverse experiences.

Source: 59 FR 54042, Oct. 27, 1994, unless otherwise noted.

(a) Definitions. The following definitions of terms apply to this section:

Adverse experience. Any adverse event associated with the use of a biological product in humans, whether or not considered product related, including the following: An adverse event occurring in the course of the use of a biological product in professional practice; an adverse event occurring from overdose of the product whether accidental or intentional; an adverse event occurring from abuse of the product; an adverse event occurring from withdrawal of the product; and any failure of expected pharmacological action.

Blood Component. As defined in Sec. 606.3(c) of this chapter.

Disability. A substantial disruption of a person's ability to conduct normal life functions.

Life-threatening adverse experience. Any adverse experience that places the patient, in the view of the initial reporter, at immediate risk of death from the adverse experience as it occurred, i.e., it does not include an adverse experience that, had it occurred in a more severe form, might have caused death.

Serious adverse experience. Any adverse experience occurring at any dose that results in any of the following outcomes: Death, a life-threatening adverse experience, inpatient hospitalization or prolongation of existing hospitalization, a persistent or significant disability/incapacity, or a congenital anomaly/birth defect. Important medical events that may not result in death, be life-threatening, or require hospitalization may be considered a serious adverse experience when, based upon appropriate medical judgment, they may jeopardize the patient or subject and may require medical or surgical intervention to prevent one of the outcomes listed in this definition. Examples of such medical events include allergic bronchospasm requiring intensive treatment in an emergency room or at home, blood dyscrasias or convulsions that do not result in inpatient hospitalization, or the development of drug dependency or drug abuse.

Unexpected adverse experience: Any adverse experience that is not listed in the current labeling for the biological product. This includes events that may be symptomatically and pathophysiologically related to an event listed in the labeling, but differ from the event because of greater severity or specificity. For example, under this definition, hepatic necrosis would be unexpected (by virtue of greater severity) if the labeling only referred to elevated hepatic enzymes or hepatitis.

Similarly, cerebral thromboembolism and cerebral vasculitis would be unexpected (by virtue of greater specificity) if the labeling only listed cerebral vascular accidents. "Unexpected," as used in this definition, refers to an adverse experience that has not been previously observed (i.e., included in the labeling) rather than from the perspective of such experience not being anticipated from the pharmacological properties of the pharmaceutical product.

(b) Review of adverse experiences. Any person having a product license under Sec. 601.20 of this chapter shall promptly review all adverse experience information pertaining to its product obtained or otherwise received by the licensed manufacturer from any source, foreign or domestic, including information derived from commercial marketing experience, postmarketing clinical investigations, postmarketing epidemiological/surveillance studies, reports in the scientific literature, and unpublished scientific papers. Licensed manufacturers are not required to resubmit to FDA adverse product experience reports forwarded to the licensed manufacturer by FDA; licensed manufacturers, however, must submit all followup information on such reports to FDA.

Any person subject to the reporting requirements under paragraph (c) of this section shall also develop written procedures for the surveillance, receipt, evaluation, and reporting of postmarketing adverse experiences to FDA.

(c) Reporting requirements. The licensed manufacturer shall report to FDA adverse experience information, as described in this section. The licensed manufacturer shall submit two copies of each report described in this section for nonvaccine biological products, to the Center for Biologics Evaluation and Research (HFM-210), Food and Drug Administration, 1401 Rockville Pike, suite 200 N., Rockville, MD 20852-1448. Submit all vaccine adverse experience reports to: Vaccine Adverse Event Reporting System (VAERS), P.O. Box 1100, Rockville, MD 20849-1100. FDA may waive the requirement for the second copy in appropriate instances.

(1)(i) Postmarketing 15-day "Alert reports". The licensed manufacturer shall report each adverse experience that is both serious and unexpected, whether foreign or domestic, as soon as possible but in no case later than 15 calendar days of initial receipt of the information by the licensed manufacturer.

(ii) Postmarketing 15-day "Alert reports"—followup. The licensed manufacturer shall promptly investigate all adverse experiences that are the subject of these postmarketing 15-day Alert reports and shall submit followup reports within 15 calendar days of receipt of new information or as requested by FDA. If additional information is not obtainable, records should be maintained of the unsuccessful steps taken to seek additional information. Postmarketing 15-day Alert reports and followups to them shall be submitted under separate cover.

(iii) Submission of reports. The requirements of paragraphs (c)(1)(i) and (c)(1)(ii) of this section, concerning the submission of postmarketing 15-day Alert reports, shall also apply to any person whose name appears on the label of a licensed biological product as a manufacturer, packer, distributor, shared manufacturer, joint manufacturer, or any other participant involved in divided manufacturing. To avoid unnecessary duplication in the submission to FDA of reports required by paragraphs (c)(1)(i) and (c)(1)(ii) of this section, obligations of persons other than the licensed manufacturer of the final biological product may be met by submission of all reports of serious adverse experiences to the licensed manufacturer of the final product. If a person elects to submit adverse experience reports to the licensed manufacturer of the final product rather than to FDA, the person shall submit each report to the licensed manufacturer of the final product within 5 calendar days of receipt of the report by the person, and the licensed manufacturer of the final product shall then comply with the requirements of this section. Under this circumstance, a person who elects to submit reports to the licensed manufacturer of the final product shall maintain a record of this action which shall include:

(A) A copy of all adverse biological product experience reports submitted to the licensed manufacturer of the final product;

(B) The date the report was received by the person;

(C) The date the report was submitted to the licensed manufacturer of the final product; and-

(D) The name and address of the licensed manufacturer of the final product.

(iv) Report identification. Each report submitted under this paragraph shall bear prominent identification as to its contents, i.e., "15-day Alert report," or "15-day Alert report-followup."

(2) Periodic adverse experience reports. (i) The licensed manufacturer shall report each adverse experience not reported under paragraph (c)(1)(i) of this section at quarterly intervals, for 3 years from the date of issuance of the product license, and then at annual intervals. The licensed manufacturer shall submit each quarterly report within 30 days of the close of the quarter (the first quarter beginning on the date of issuance of the product license) and each annual report within 60 days of the anniversary date of the issuance of the product license. Upon written notice, FDA may extend or reestablish the requirement that a licensed manufacturer submit quarterly reports, or require that the licensed manufacturer submit reports under this section at different times than those stated. Followup information to adverse experiences submitted in a periodic report may be submitted in the next periodic report.

(ii) Each periodic report shall contain:

(A) A narrative summary and analysis of the information in the report and an analysis of the 15-day Alert reports submitted during the reporting interval (all 15-day Alert reports being appropriately referenced by the licensed manufacturer's patient identification number, adverse reaction term(s), and date of submission to FDA);

(B) A form designated for Adverse Experience Reporting by FDA for each adverse experience not reported under paragraph (c)(1)(i) of this section (with an index consisting of a line listing of the licensed manufacturer's patient identification number and adverse reaction term(s)); and

(C) A history of actions taken since the last report because of adverse experiences (for example, labeling changes or studies initiated).

(iii) Periodic reporting, except for information regarding 15-day Alert reports, does not apply to adverse experience information obtained from postmarketing studies (whether or not conducted under an investigational new drug application), from reports in the scientific literature, and from foreign marketing experience.

(d) Scientific literature. (1) A 15-day Alert report based on information from the scientific literature shall be accompanied by a copy of the published article. The 15-day Alert reporting requirements in paragraph (c)(1)(i) of this section (i.e., serious, unexpected adverse experiences) apply only to reports found in scientific and medical journals either as case reports or as the result of a formal clinical trial.

(2) As with all reports submitted under paragraph (c)(1)(i) of this section, reports based on the scientific literature shall be submitted on the reporting form designated by FDA or comparable format as prescribed by paragraph (f) of this section. In cases where the licensed manufacturer believes that preparing the form designated by FDA constitutes an undue hardship, the licensed manufacturer may arrange with the Division of Biostatistics and Epidemiology (HFM-210) for an acceptable alternative reporting format.

(e) Postmarketing studies. (1) Licensed manufacturers are not required to submit a 15-day Alert report under paragraph (c) of this section for an adverse experience obtained from a postmarketing clinical study (whether or not conducted under a biological investigational new drug application) unless the licensed manufacturer concludes that there is a reasonable possibility that the product caused the adverse experience.

(2) The licensed manufacturer shall separate and clearly mark reports of adverse experiences that occur during a postmarketing study as being distinct from those experiences that are being reported spontaneously to the licensed manufacturer.

(f) Reporting forms. (1) Except as provided in paragraph (f)(3) of this section, the licensed manufacturer shall complete the reporting form designated by FDA for each report of an adverse experience (FDA Form 3500A, or, for vaccines, a VAERS form; foreign events including those associated with the use of vaccines, may be submitted either on an FDA Form 3500A or, if preferred, on a CIOMS I form).

(2) Each completed form should refer only to an individual patient or single attached publication.

(3) Instead of using a designated reporting form, a licensed manufacturer may use a computer-generated form or other alternative format (e.g., a computer-generated tape or tabular listing) provided that:

(i) The content of the alternative format is equivalent in all elements of information to those specified in the form designated by FDA; and

(ii) the format is approved in advance by MEDWATCH: The FDA Medical Products Reporting Program; or, for alternatives to the VAERS Form, by the Division of Biostatistics and Epidemiology.

(4) Copies of the reporting form designated by FDA (FDA-3500A) for nonvaccine biological products may be obtained from the Center for Biologics Evaluation and Research (address above). Additional supplies of the form may be obtained from the Consolidated Forms and Publications Distribution Center, 3222 Hubbard Rd., Landover, MD 20785. Supplies of the VAERS form may be obtained from VAERS by calling 1-800-822-7967.

(g)Multiple reports. A licensed manufacturer should not include in reports under this section any adverse experience that occurred in clinical trials if they were previously submitted as part of the license application. If a report refers to more than one biological product marketed by a licensed manufacturer, the licensed manufacturer should submit the report to the license for the product listed first in the report.

(h) *Patient privacy.* For nonvaccine biological products, a licensed manufacturer should not include in reports under this section the names and addresses of individual patients; instead, the licensed manufacturer should assign a unique code number to each report, preferably not more than eight characters in length. The licensed manufacturer should include the name of the reporter from whom the information was received. The names of patients, health care professionals, hospitals, and geographical identifiers in adverse experience reports are not releasable to the public under FDA's public information regulations in part 20 this of chapter. For vaccine adverse experience reports, these data will become part of the CDC Privacy Act System 09-20-0136, "Epidemiologic Studies and Surveillance of Disease Problems." Information identifying the person who received the vaccine or that person's legal representative will not be made available to the public, but may be available to the vaccinee or legal representative.

(i) *Recordkeeping.* The licensed manufacturer shall maintain for a period of 10 years records of all adverse experiences known to the licensed manufacturer, including raw data and any correspondence relating to the adverse experiences.

(j) *Revocation of license.* If a licensed manufacturer fails to establish and maintain records and make reports required under this section with respect to a licensed biological product, FDA may revoke the product license for such a product in accordance with the procedures of Sec. 601.5 of this chapter.

(k) *Exemptions.* Manufacturers of the following listed products are not required to submit adverse experience reports under this section:

(1) Whole blood or components of whole blood.

(2) In vitro diagnostic products, including assay systems for the detection of antibodies or antigens to retroviruses. These products are subject to the reporting requirements for devices.

(l) *Disclaimer.* A report or information submitted by a licensed manufacturer under this section (and any release by FDA of that report or information) does not necessarily reflect a conclusion by the licensed manufacturer or FDA that the report or information constitutes an admission that the biological product caused or contributed to an adverse effect. A licensed manufacturer need not admit, and may deny, that the report or information submitted under this section constitutes an admission that the biological product caused or contributed to an adverse effect. For purposes of this provision, this paragraph also includes any person reporting under paragraph (c)(1)(iii) of this section.

[59 FR 54042, Oct. 27, 1994, as amended at 62 FR 34168, June 25, 1997; 62 FR 52252, Oct. 7, 1997; 63 FR 14612, Mar. 26, 1998]

Effective Date Note: At 62 FR 52252, Oct. 7, 1997, Sec. 600.80 was amended by revising paragraphs (a), (c)(1), (f)(1), and the first sentence of paragraph (g); by adding two new sentences at the end of paragraph (b); and by removing paragraph (j) and redesignating paragraphs (k), (l), and (m) as paragraphs (j), (k), and (l), respectively, effective Apr. 6, 1998. At 63 FR 14612, Mar. 26, 1998, the last sentence of paragraph (l) was corrected by revising "(c)(1)(ii)" to read "(c)(1)(iii)", effective April 6, 1998.

Sec. 600.81 Distribution reports.

The licensed manufacturer shall submit information about the quantity of the product distributed under the product license, including the quantity distributed to distributors. The interval between distribution reports shall be 6 months. Upon written notice, FDA may require that the licensed manufacturer submit distribution reports under this section at times other than every 6 months. The distribution report shall consist of the bulk lot number (from which the final container was filled), the fill lot numbers for the total number of dosage units of each strength or potency distributed (e.g., fifty thousand per 10-milliliter vials), the label lot number (if different from fill lot number), labeled date of expiration, number of doses in fill lot/label lot, date of release of fill lot/label lot for distribution at that time. If any significant amount of a fill lot/label lot is returned, include this information. Disclosure of financial or pricing data is not required. As needed, FDA may require submission of more detailed product distribution information. Upon written notice, FDA may require that the licensed manufacturer submit reports under this section at times other than those stated. Requests by a licensed manufacturer to submit reports at times other than those stated should be made as a request for a waiver under Sec. 600.90.

Sec. 600.90 Waivers.

(a) A licensed manufacturer may ask the Food and Drug Administration to waive under this section any requirement that applies to the licensed manufacturer under Secs. 600.80 and 600.81. A waiver request under this section is required to be submitted with supporting documentation. The waiver request is required to contain one of the following:

(1) An explanation why the licensed manufacturer's compliance with the requirement is unnecessary or cannot be achieved,

(2) A description of an alternative submission that satisfies the purpose of the requirement, or

(3) Other information justifying a waiver.

(b) FDA may grant a waiver if it finds one of the following:

(1) The licensed manufacturer's compliance with the requirement is unnecessary or cannot be achieved,

(2) The licensed manufacturer's alternative submission satisfies the requirement, or

(3) The licensed manufacturer's submission otherwise justifies a waiver.

PART 812—INVESTIGATIONAL DEVICE EXEMPTIONS

Subpart A—General Provisions

Sec. 812.1 Scope.

(a) The purpose of this part is to encourage, to the extent consistent with the protection of public health and safety and with ethical standards, the discovery and development of useful devices intended for human use, and to that end to maintain optimum freedom for scientific investigators in their pursuit of this purpose. This part provides procedures for the conduct of clinical investigations of devices. An approved investigational device exemption (IDE) permits a device that otherwise would be required to comply with a performance standard or to have premarket approval to be shipped lawfully for the purpose of conducting investigations of that device. An IDE approved under Sec. 812.30 or considered approved under Sec. 812.2(b) exempts a device from the requirements of the following sections of the Federal Food, Drug, and Cosmetic Act (the act) and regulations issued thereunder: Misbranding under section 502 of the act, registration, listing, and premarket notification under section 510, performance standards under section 514, premarket approval under section 515, a banned device regulation under section 516, records and reports under section 519, restricted device requirements under section 520(e), good manufacturing practice requirements under section 520(f) except for the requirements found in Sec. 820.30, if applicable (unless the sponsor states an intention to comply with these requirements under Sec. 812.20(b)(3) or Sec. 812.140(b)(4)(v)) and color additive requirements under section 721.

(b) References in this part to regulatory sections of the Code of Federal Regulations are to chapter I of title 21, unless otherwise noted.

[45 FR 3751, Jan. 18, 1980, as amended at 59 FR 14366, Mar. 28, 1994; 61 FR 52654, Oct. 7, 1996]

Sec. 812.2 Applicability.

(a) *General.* This part applies to all clinical investigations of devices to determine safety and effectiveness, except as provided in paragraph (c) of this section.

(b) *Abbreviated requirements.* The following categories of investigations are considered to have approved applications for IDE's, unless FDA has notified a sponsor under Sec. 812.20(a) that approval of an application is required:

(1) An investigation of a device other than a significant risk device, if the device is not a banned device and the sponsor:

(i) Labels the device in accordance with Sec. 812.5;

(ii) Obtains IRB approval of the investigation after presenting the reviewing IRB with a brief explanation of why the device is not a significant risk device, and maintains such approval;

(iii) Ensures that each investigator participating in an investigation of the device obtains from each subject under the investigator's care, informed consent under part 50 and documents it, unless documentation is waived by an IRB under Sec. 56.109(c).

(iv) Complies with the requirements of Sec. 812.46 with respect to monitoring investigations;

(v) Maintains the records required under Sec. 812.140(b) (4) and (5) and makes the reports required under Sec. 812.150(b) (1) through (3) and

(5) through (10);

(vi) Ensures that participating investigators maintain the records required by Sec. 812.140(a)(3)(i) and make the reports required under Sec. 812.150(a) (1), (2), (5), and (7); and

(vii) Complies with the prohibitions in Sec. 812.7 against promotion and other practices.

(2) An investigation of a device other than one subject to paragraph (e) of this section, if the investigation was begun on or before July 16, 1980, and to be completed, and is completed, on or before January 19, 1981.

(c) Exempted investigations. This part, with the exception of Sec. 812.119, does not apply to investigations of the following categories of devices:

(1) A device, other than a transitional device, in commercial distribution immediately before May 28, 1976, when used or investigated in accordance with the indications in labeling in effect at that time.

(2) A device, other than a transitional device, introduced into commercial distribution on or after May 28, 1976, that FDA has determined to be substantially equivalent to a device in commercial distribution immediately before May 28, 1976, and that is used or investigated in accordance with the indications in the labeling FDA reviewed under subpart E of part 807 in determining substantial equivalence.

(3) A diagnostic device, if the sponsor complies with applicable requirements in Sec. 809.10(c) and if the testing:

(i) Is noninvasive,

(ii) Does not require an invasive sampling procedure that presents significant risk,

(iii) Does not by design or intention introduce energy into a subject, and

(iv) Is not used as a diagnostic procedure without confirmation of the diagnosis by another, medically established diagnostic product or procedure.

(4) A device undergoing consumer preference testing, testing of a modification, or testing of a combination of two or more devices in commercial distribution, if the testing is not for the purpose of determining safety or effectiveness and does not put subjects at risk.

(5) A device intended solely for veterinary use.

(6) A device shipped solely for research on or with laboratory animals and labeled in accordance with Sec. 812.5(c).

(7) A custom device as defined in Sec. 812.3(b), unless the device is being used to determine safety or effectiveness for commercial distribution.

(d) Limit on certain exemptions. In the case of class II or class III device described in paragraph (c)(1) or (2) of this section, this part applies beginning on the date stipulated in an FDA regulation or order that calls for the submission of premarket approval applications for an unapproved class III device, or establishes a performance standard for a class II device.

(e) Investigations subject to IND's. A sponsor that, on July 16, 1980, has an effective investigational new drug application (IND) for an investigation of a device shall continue to comply with the requirements of part 312 until 90 days after that date. To continue the investigation after that date, a sponsor shall comply with paragraph (b)(1) of this section, if the device is not a significant risk device, or shall have obtained FDA approval under Sec. 812.30 of an IDE application for the investigation of the device.

[45 FR 3751, Jan. 18, 1980, as amended at 46 FR 8956, Jan. 27, 1981; 46 FR 14340, Feb. 27, 1981; 53 FR 11252, Apr. 6, 1988; 62 FR 4165, Jan, 29, 1997; 62 FR 12096, Mar. 14, 1997]

Sec. 812.3 Definitions.

(a) Act means the Federal Food, Drug, and Cosmetic Act (sections 201-901, 52 Stat. 1040 et seq., as amended (21 U.S.C. 301-392)).

(b) Custom device means a device that:

(1) Necessarily deviates from devices generally available or from an applicable performance standard or premarket approval requirement in order to comply with the order of an individual physician or dentist;

(2) Is not generally available to, or generally used by, other physicians or dentists;

(3) Is not generally available in finished form for purchase or for dispensing upon prescription;

(4) Is not offered for commercial distribution through labeling or advertising; and

(5) Is intended for use by an individual patient named in the order of a physician or dentist, and is to be made in a specific form for that patient, or is intended to meet the special needs of the physician or dentist in the course of professional practice.

(c) FDA means the Food and Drug Administration.

(d) Implant means a device that is placed into a surgically or naturally formed cavity of the human body if it is intended to remain there for a period of 30 days or more. FDA may, in order to protect public health, determine that devices placed in subjects for shorter periods are also "implants" for purposes of this part.

(e) Institution means a person, other than an individual, who engages in the conduct of research on subjects or in the delivery of medical services to individuals as a primary activity or as an adjunct to providing residential or custodial care to humans. The term includes, for example, a hospital, retirement home, confinement facility, academic establishment, and device manufacturer. The term has the same meaning as "facility" in section 520(g) of the act.

(f) Institutional review board (IRB) means any board, committee, or other group formally designated by an institution to review biomedical research involving subjects and established, operated, and functioning in conformance with part 56. The term has the same meaning as "institutional review committee" in section 520(g) of the act.

(g) Investigational device means a device, including a transitional device, that is the object of an investigation.

(h) Investigation means a clinical investigation or research involving one or more subjects to determine the safety or effectiveness of a device.

(i) Investigator means an individual who actually conducts a clinical investigation, i.e., under whose immediate direction the test article is administered or dispensed to, or used involving, a subject, or, in the event of an investigation conducted by a team of individuals, is the responsible leader of that team.

(j) Monitor, when used as a noun, means an individual designated by a sponsor or contract research organization to oversee the progress of an investigation. The monitor may be an employee of a sponsor or a consultant to the sponsor, or an employee of or consultant to a contract research organization. Monitor, when used as a verb, means to oversee an investigation.

(k) Noninvasive, when applied to a diagnostic device or procedure, means one that does not by design or intention: (1) Penetrate or pierce the skin or mucous membranes of the body, the ocular cavity, or the urethra, or (2) enter the ear beyond the external auditory canal, the nose beyond the nares, the mouth beyond the pharynx, the anal canal beyond the rectum, or the vagina beyond the cervical os. For purposes of this part, blood sampling that involves simple venipuncture is considered noninvasive, and the use of surplus samples of body fluids or tissues that are left over from samples taken for noninvestigational purposes is also considered noninvasive.

(l) Person includes any individual, partnership, corporation, association, scientific or academic establishment, Government agency or organizational unit of a Government agency, and any other legal entity.

(m) Significant risk device means an investigational device that:

(1) Is intended as an implant and presents a potential for serious risk to the health, safety, or welfare of a subject;

(2) Is purported or represented to be for a use in supporting or sustaining human life and presents a potential for serious risk to the health, safety, or welfare of a subject;

(3) Is for a use of substantial importance in diagnosing, curing, mitigating, or treating disease, or otherwise preventing impairment of human health and presents a potential for serious risk to the health, safety, or welfare of a subject; or

(4) Otherwise presents a potential for serious risk to the health, safety, or welfare of a subject.

(n) Sponsor means a person who initiates, but who does not actually conduct, the investigation, that is, the investigational device is administered, dispensed, or used under the immediate direction of another individual. A person other than an individual that uses one or more of its own employees to conduct an investigation that it has initiated is a sponsor, not a sponsor-investigator, and the employees are investigators.

(o) Sponsor-investigator means an individual who both initiates and actually conducts, alone or with others, an investigation, that is, under whose immediate direction the investigational device is administered, dispensed, or used. The term does not include any person other than an individual. The obligations of a sponsor-investigator under this part include those of an investigator and those of a sponsor.

(p) Subject means a human who participates in an investigation, either as an individual on whom or on whose specimen an investigational device is used or as a control. A subject may be in normal health or may have a medical condition or disease.

(q) Termination means a discontinuance, by sponsor or by withdrawal of IRB or FDA approval, of an investigation before completion.

(r) Transitional device means a device subject to section 520(l) of the act, that is, a device that FDA considered to be a new drug or an antibiotic drug before May 28, 1976.

(s) Unanticipated adverse device effect means any serious adverse effect on health or safety or any life-threatening problem or death caused by, or associated with, a device, if that effect, problem, or death was not previously identified in nature, severity, or degree of incidence in the investigational plan or application (including a supplementary plan or application), or any other unanticipated serious problem associated with a device that relates to the rights, safety, or welfare of subjects.

[45 FR 3751, Jan. 18, 1980, as amended at 46 FR 8956, Jan. 27, 1981; 48 FR 15622, Apr. 12, 1983]

Sec. 812.5 Labeling of investigational devices.

(a) Contents. An investigational device or its immediate package shall bear a label with the following information: the name and place of business of the manufacturer, packer, or distributor (in accordance with Sec. 801.1), the quantity of contents, if appropriate, and the following statement:

"CAUTION—Investigational device. Limited by Federal (or United States) law to investigational use." The label or other labeling shall describe all relevant contraindications, hazards, adverse effects, interfering substances or devices, warnings, and precautions.

(b) Prohibitions. The labeling of an investigational device shall not bear any statement that is false or misleading in any particular and shall not represent that the device is safe or effective for the purposes for which it is being investigated.

(c) Animal research. An investigational device shipped solely for research on or with laboratory animals shall bear on its label the following statement: "CAUTION—Device for investigational use in laboratory animals or other tests that do not involve human subjects."

[45 FR 3751, Jan. 18, 1980, as amended at 45 FR 58842, Sept. 5, 1980]

Sec. 812.7 Prohibition of promotion and other practices.

A sponsor, investigator, or any person acting for or on behalf of a sponsor or investigator shall not:

(a) Promote or test market an investigational device, until after FDA has approved the device for commercial distribution.

(b) Commercialize an investigational device by charging the subjects or investigators for a device a price larger than that necessary to recover costs of manufacture, research, development, and handling.

(c) Unduly prolong an investigation. If data developed by the investigation indicate in the case of a class III device that premarket approval cannot be justified or in the case of a class II device that it will not comply with an applicable performance standard or an amendment to that standard, the sponsor shall promptly terminate the investigation.

(d) Represent that an investigational device is safe or effective for the purposes for which it is being investigated.

Sec. 812.10 Waivers.

(a) Request. A sponsor may request FDA to waive any requirement of this part. A waiver request, with supporting documentation, may be submitted separately or as part of an application to the address in Sec. 812.19.

(b) FDA action. FDA may by letter grant a waiver of any requirement that FDA finds is not required by the act and is unnecessary to protect the rights, safety, or welfare of human subjects.

(c) Effect of request. Any requirement shall continue to apply unless and until FDA waives it.

Sec. 812.18 Import and export requirements.

(a) Imports. In addition to complying with other requirements of this part, a person who imports or offers for importation an investigational device subject to this part shall be the agent of the foreign exporter with respect to investigations of the device and shall act as the sponsor of the clinical investigation, or ensure that another person acts as the agent of the foreign exporter and the sponsor of the investigation.

(b) Exports. A person exporting an investigational device subject to this part shall obtain FDA's prior approval, as required by section 801(e) of the act or comply with section 802 of the act.

[45 FR 3751, Jan. 18, 1980, as amended at 62 FR 26229, May 13, 1997]

Sec. 812.19 Address for IDE correspondence.

All applications, supplemental applications, reports, requests for waivers, requests for import or export approval, and other correspondence relating to matters covered by this part shall be addressed to the Center for Devices and Radiological Health, Document Mail Center (HFZ-401), Food and Drug Administration, 1390 Piccard Dr., Rockville, MD 20850. The outside wrapper of each submission shall state what the submission is, for example an "IDE application," a "supplemental IDE application," or "correspondence concerning an IDE (or an IDE application)."

[45 FR 3751, Jan. 18, 1980, as amended at 53 FR 11252, Apr. 6, 1988; 55 FR 11169, Mar. 27, 1990]

Subpart B—Application and Administrative Action

Sec. 812.20 Application.

(a) Submission. (1) A sponsor shall submit an application to FDA if the sponsor intends to use a significant risk device in an investigation, intends to conduct an investigation that involves an exception from informed consent under Sec. 50.24 of this chapter, or if FDA notifies the sponsor that an application is required for an investigation.

(2) A sponsor shall not begin an investigation for which FDA's approval of an application is required until FDA has approved the application.

(3) A sponsor shall submit three copies of a signed "Application for an Investigational Device Exemption" (IDE application), together with accompanying materials, by registered mail or by hand to the address in Sec. 812.19. Subsequent correspondence concerning an application or a supplemental application shall be submitted by registered mail or by hand.

(4)(i) A sponsor shall submit a separate IDE for any clinical investigation involving an exception from informed consent under Sec. 50.24 of this chapter. Such a clinical investigation is not permitted to proceed without the prior written authorization of FDA. FDA shall provide such written authorization 30 days after FDA receives the IDE or earlier.

(ii) If the investigation involves an exception from informed consent under Sec. 50.24 of this chapter, the sponsor shall prominently identify on the cover sheet that the investigation is subject to the requirements in Sec. 50.24 of this chapter.

(b) Contents. An IDE application shall include, in the following order:

(1) The name and address of the sponsor.

(2) A complete report of prior investigations of the device and an accurate summary of those sections of the investigational plan described in Sec. 812.25(a) through (e) or, in lieu of the summary, the complete plan. The sponsor shall submit to FDA a complete investigational plan and a complete report of prior investigations of the device if no IRB has reviewed them, if FDA has found an IRB's review inadequate, or if FDA requests them.

(3) A description of the methods, facilities, and controls used for the manufacture, processing, packing, storage, and, where appropriate, installation of the device, in sufficient detail so that a person generally familiar with good manufacturing practices can make a knowledgeable judgment about the quality control used in the manufacture of the device.

(4) An example of the agreements to be entered into by all investigators to comply with investigator obligations under this part, and a list of the names and addresses of all investigators who have signed the agreement.

(5) A certification that all investigators who will participate in the investigation have signed the agreement, that the list of investigators includes all the investigators participating in the investigation, and that no investigators will be added to the investigation until they have signed the agreement.

(6) A list of the name, address, and chairperson of each IRB that has been or will be asked to review the investigation and a certification of the action concerning the investigation taken by each such IRB.

(7) The name and address of any institution at which a part of the investigation may be conducted that has not been identified in accordance with paragraph (b)(6) of this section.

(8) If the device is to be sold, the amount to be charged and an explanation of why sale does not constitute commercialization of the device.

(9) A claim for categorical exclusion under Sec. 25.30 or 25.34 or an environmental assessment under Sec. 25.40.

(10) Copies of all labeling for the device.

(11) Copies of all forms and informational materials to be provided to subjects to obtain informed consent.

(12) Any other relevant information FDA requests for review of the application.

(c) Additional information. FDA may request additional information concerning an investigation or revision in the investigational plan. The sponsor may treat such a request as a disapproval of the application for purposes of requesting a hearing under part 16.

(d) Information previously submitted. Information previously submitted to the Center for Devices and Radiological Health in accordance with this chapter ordinarily need not be resubmitted, but may be incorporated by reference.

[45 FR 3751, Jan. 18, 1980, as amended at 46 FR 8956, Jan. 27, 1981; 50 FR 16669, Apr. 26, 1985; 53 FR 11252, Apr. 6, 1988; 61 FR 51530, Oct. 2, 1996; 62 FR 40600, July 29, 1997]

Sec. 812.25 Investigational plan.

The investigational plan shall include, in the following order:

(a) Purpose. The name and intended use of the device and the objectives and duration of the investigation.

(b) Protocol. A written protocol describing the methodology to be used and an analysis of the protocol demonstrating that the investigation is scientifically sound.

(c) Risk analysis. A description and analysis of all increased risks to which subjects will be exposed by the investigation; the manner in which these risks will be minimized; a justification for the investigation; and a description of the patient population, including the number, age, sex, and condition.

(d) *Description of device.* A description of each important component, ingredient, property, and principle of operation of the device and of each anticipated change in the device during the course of the investigation.

(e) *Monitoring procedures.* The sponsor's written procedures for monitoring the investigation and the name and address of any monitor.

(f) *Labeling.* Copies of all labeling for the device.

(g) *Consent materials.* Copies of all forms and informational materials to be provided to subjects to obtain informed consent.

(h) *IRB information.* A list of the names, locations, and chairpersons of all IRB's that have been or will be asked to review the investigation, and a certification of any action taken by any of those IRB's with respect to the investigation.

(i) *Other institutions.* The name and address of each institution at which a part of the investigation may be conducted that has not been identified in paragraph (h) of this section.

(j) *Additional records and reports.* A description of records and reports that will be maintained on the investigation in addition to those prescribed in subpart G.

Sec. 812.27 Report of prior investigations.

(a) *General.* The report of prior investigations shall include reports of all prior clinical, animal, and laboratory testing of the device and shall be comprehensive and adequate to justify the proposed investigation.

(b) *Specific contents.* The report also shall include:

(1) A bibliography of all publications, whether adverse or supportive, that are relevant to an evaluation of the safety or effectiveness of the device, copies of all published and unpublished adverse information, and, if requested by an IRB or FDA, copies of other significant publications.

(2) A summary of all other unpublished information (whether adverse or supportive) in the possession of, or reasonably obtainable by, the sponsor that is relevant to an evaluation of the safety or effectiveness of the device.

(3) If information on nonclinical laboratory studies is provided, a statement that all such studies have been conducted in compliance with applicable requirements in the good laboratory practice regulations in part 58, or if any such study was not conducted in compliance with such regulations, a brief statement of the reason for the noncompliance. Failure or inability to comply with this requirement does not justify failure to provide information on a relevant nonclinical test study.

[45 FR 3751, Jan. 18, 1980, as amended at 50 FR 7518, Feb. 22, 1985]

Sec. 812.30 FDA action on applications.

(a) *Approval or disapproval.* FDA will notify the sponsor in writing of the date it receives an application. FDA may approve an investigation as proposed, approve it with modifications, or disapprove it. An investigation may not begin until:

(1) Thirty days after FDA receives the application at the address in Sec. 812.19 for the investigation of a device other than a banned device, unless FDA notifies the sponsor that the investigation may not begin; or

(2) FDA approves, by order, an IDE for the investigation.

(b) *Grounds for disapproval or withdrawal.* FDA may disapprove or withdraw approval of an application if FDA finds that:

(1) There has been a failure to comply with any requirement of this part or the act, any other applicable regulation or statute, or any condition of approval imposed by an IRB or FDA.

(2) The application or a report contains an untrue statement of a material fact, or omits material information required by this part.

(3) The sponsor fails to respond to a request for additional information within the time

prescribed by FDA.

(4) There is reason to believe that the risks to the subjects are not outweighed by the anticipated benefits to the subjects and the importance of the knowledge to be gained, or informed consent is inadquate, or the investigation is scientifically unsound, or there is reason to believe that the device as used is ineffective.

(5) It is otherwise unreasonable to begin or to continue the investigation owing to the way in which the device is used or the inadequacy of:

(i) The report of prior investigations or the investigational plan;

(ii) The methods, facilities, and controls used for the manufacturing, processing, packaging, storage, and, where appropriate, installation of the device; or

(iii) Monitoring and review of the investigation.

(c) Notice of disapproval or withdrawal. If FDA disapproves an application or proposes to withdraw approval of an application, FDA will notify the sponsor in writing.

(1) A disapproval order will contain a complete statement of the reasons for disapproval and a statement that the sponsor has an opportunity to request a hearing under part 16.

(2) A notice of a proposed withdrawal of approval will contain a complete statement of the reasons for withdrawal and a statement that the sponsor has an opportunity to request a hearing under part 16. FDA will provide the opportunity for hearing before withdrawal of approval, unless FDA determines in the notice that continuation of testing under the exemption will result in an unreasonable risk to the public health and orders withdrawal of approval before any hearing.

[45 FR 3751, Jan. 18, 1980, as amended at 45 FR 58842, Sept. 5, 1980]

Sec. 812.35 Supplemental applications.

(a) Changes in investigational plan. A sponsor shall: (1) Submit to FDA a supplemental application if the sponsor or an investigator proposes a change in the investigational plan that may affect its scientific soundness or the rights, safety, or welfare of subjects, and (2) obtain FDA approval under Sec. 812.30(a) of any such change, and IRB approval when the change involves the rights, safety, or welfare of subjects (see Secs. 56.110 and 56.111), before implementation. These requirements do not apply in the case of a deviation from the investigational plan to protect the life or physical well-being of a subject in an emergency, which deviation shall be reported to FDA within 5 working days after the sponsor learns of it (see Sec. 812.150(a)(4)).

Whenever a sponsor intends to conduct a clinical investigation with an exception from informed consent for emergency research as set forth in Sec. 50.24 of this chapter, the sponsor shall submit a separate IDE for such investigation.

(b) IRB approval for new facilities. A sponsor shall submit to FDA a certification of any IRB approval of an investigation or a part of an investigation not included in the IDE application. If the investigation is otherwise unchanged, the supplemental application shall consist of an updating of the information required by Sec. 812.20(b) and (c) and a description of any modifications in the investigational plan required by the IRB as a condition of approval. A certification of IRB approval need not be included in the initial submission of the supplemental application, and such certification is not a precondition for agency consideration of the application. Nevertheless, a sponsor may not begin a part of an investigation at a facility until the IRB has approved the investigation, FDA has received the certification of IRB approval, and FDA, under Sec. 812.30(a), has approved the supplemental application relating to that part of the investigation (see Sec. 56.103(a)).

[50 FR 25909, June 24, 1985; 50 FR 28932, July 17, 1985; 61 FR 51531, Oct. 2, 1996]

Sec. 812.36 Treatment use of an investigational device.

(a) General. A device that is not approved for marketing may be under clinical investigation for a serious or immediately life-threatening disease or condition in patients for whom no comparable or satisfactory alternative device or other therapy is available. During the clinical trial or prior to final action on the marketing application, it may be appropriate to use the device in the treatment of patients not in the trial under the provisions of a treatment investigational device exemption (IDE). The purpose of this section is to facilitate the availability of promising new devices to desperately ill patients as early in the device development process as possible, before general marketing begins, and to obtain additional data on the device's safety and effectiveness. In the case of a serious disease, a device ordinarily may be made available for treatment use under this section after all clinical trials have been completed. In the case of an immediately life-threatening disease, a device may be made available for treatment use under this section prior to the completion of all clinical trials. For the purpose of this section, an "immediately life-threatening" disease means a stage of a disease in which there is a reasonable likelihood that death will occur within a matter of months or in which premature death is likely without early treatment. For purposes of this section, "treatment use" of a device includes the use of a device for diagnostic purposes.

(b) Criteria. FDA shall consider the use of an investigational device under a treatment IDE if:

(1) The device is intended to treat or diagnose a serious or immediately life-threatening disease or condition;

(2) There is no comparable or satisfactory alternative device or other therapy available to treat or diagnose that stage of the disease or condition in the intended patient population;

(3) The device is under investigation in a controlled clinical trial for the same use under an approved IDE, or such clinical trials have been completed; and

(4) The sponsor of the investigation is actively pursuing marketing approval/clearance of the investigational device with due diligence.

(c) Applications for treatment use. (1) A treatment IDE application shall include, in the following order:

(i) The name, address, and telephone number of the sponsor of the treatment IDE;

(ii) The intended use of the device, the criteria for patient selection, and a written protocol describing the treatment use;

(iii) An explanation of the rationale for use of the device, including, as appropriate, either a list of the available regimens that ordinarily should be tried before using the investigational device or an explanation of why the use of the investigational device is preferable to the use of available marketed treatments;

(iv) A description of clinical procedures, laboratory tests, or other measures that will be used to evaluate the effects of the device and to minimize risk;

(v) Written procedures for monitoring the treatment use and the name and address of the monitor;

(vi) Instructions for use for the device and all other labeling as required under Sec. 812.5(a) and (b);

(vii) Information that is relevant to the safety and effectiveness of the device for the intended treatment use. Information from other IDE's may be incorporated by reference to support the treatment use;

(viii) A statement of the sponsor's commitment to meet all applicable responsibilities under this part and part 56 of this chapter and to ensure compliance of all participating investigators with the informed consent requirements of part 50 of this chapter;

(ix) An example of the agreement to be signed by all investigators participating in the treatment IDE and certification that no investigator will be added to the treatment IDE before the agreement is signed; and

(x) If the device is to be sold, the price to be charged and a statement indicating that the price is based on manufacturing and handling costs only.

(2) A licensed practitioner who receives an investigational device for treatment use under a treatment IDE is an "investigator" under the IDE and is responsible for meeting all applicable investigator responsibilities under this part and parts 50 and 56 of this chapter.

(d) FDA action on treatment IDE applications. (1) Approval of treatment IDE's. Treatment use may begin 30 days after FDA receives the treatment IDE submission at the address specified in Sec. 812.19, unless FDA notifies the sponsor in writing earlier than the 30 days that the treatment use may or may not begin. FDA may approve the treatment use as proposed or approve it with modifications.

(2) Disapproval or withdrawal of approval of treatment IDE's. FDA may disapprove or withdraw approval of a treatment IDE if:(i) The criteria specified in Sec. 812.36(b) are not met or the treatment IDE does not contain the information required in Sec. 812.36(c);

(ii) FDA determines that any of the grounds for disapproval or withdrawal of approval listed in Sec. 812.30(b)(1) through (b)(5) apply;

(iii) The device is intended for a serious disease or condition and there is insufficient evidence of safety and effectiveness to support such use;

(iv) The device is intended for an immediately life-threatening disease or condition and the available scientific evidence, taken as a whole, fails to provide a reasonable basis for concluding that the device:

(A) May be effective for its intended use in its intended population; or

(B) Would not expose the patients to whom the device is to be administered to an unreasonable and significant additional risk of illness or injury;

(v) There is reasonable evidence that the treatment use is impeding enrollment in, or otherwise interfering with the conduct or completion of, a controlled investigation of the same or another investigational device;

(vi) The device has received marketing approval/clearance or a comparable device or therapy becomes available to treat or diagnose the same indication in the same patient population for which the investigational device is being used;

(vii) The sponsor of the controlled clinical trial is not pursuing marketing approval/clearance with due diligence;

(viii) Approval of the IDE for the controlled clinical investigation of the device has been withdrawn; or

(ix) The clinical investigator(s) named in the treatment IDE are not qualified by reason of their scientific training and/or experience to use the investigational device for the intended treatment use.

(3) Notice of disapproval or withdrawal. If FDA disapproves or proposes to withdraw approval of a treatment IDE, FDA will follow the procedures set forth in Sec. 812.30(c).

(e) Safeguards. Treatment use of an investigational device is conditioned upon the sponsor and investigators complying with the safeguards of the IDE process and the regulations governing informed consent (part 50 of this chapter) and institutional review boards (part 56 of this chapter).

(f) Reporting requirements. The sponsor of a treatment IDE shall submit progress reports on a semi-annual basis to all reviewing IRB's and FDA until the filing of a marketing application. These reports shall be based on the period of time since initial approval of the treatment IDE and shall include the number of patients treated with the device under the treatment IDE, the names of the investigators participating in the treatment IDE, and a brief description of the sponsor's efforts to pursue marketing approval/clearance of the device. Upon filing of a marketing application, progress reports shall be submitted annually in accordance with Sec. 812.150(b)(5). The sponsor of a treatment IDE is responsible for submitting all other reports required under Sec. 812.150.

[62 FR 48947, Sept. 18, 1997]

Sec. 812.38 Confidentiality of data and information.

(a) Existence of IDE. FDA will not disclose the existence of an IDE unless its existence has previously been publicly disclosed or acknowledged, until FDA approves an application for premarket approval of the device subject to the IDE; or a notice of completion of a product development protocol for the device has become effective.

(b) Availability of summaries or data. (1) FDA will make publicly available, upon request, a detailed summary of information concerning the safety and effectiveness of the device that was the basis for an order approving, disapproving, or withdrawing approval of an application for an IDE for a banned device. The summary shall include information on any adverse effect on health caused by the device.

(2) If a device is a banned device or if the existence of an IDE has been publicly disclosed or acknowledged, data or information contained in the file is not available for public disclosure before approval of an application for premarket approval or the effective date of a notice of completion of a product development protocol except as provided in this section. FDA may, in its discretion, disclose a summary of selected portions of the safety and effectiveness data, that is, clinical, animal, or laboratory studies and tests of the device, for public consideration of a specific pending issue.

(3) If the existence of an IDE file has not been publicly disclosed or acknowledged, no data or information in the file are available for public disclosure except as provided in paragraphs (b)(1) and (c) of this section.

(4) Notwithstanding paragraph (b)(2) of this section, FDA will make available to the public, upon request, the information in the IDE that was required to be filed in Docket Number 95S-0158 in the Dockets Management Branch (HFA-305), Food and Drug Administration, 12420 Parklawn Dr., rm. 1-23, Rockville, MD 20857, for investigations involving an exception from informed consent under Sec. 50.24 of this chapter. Persons wishing to request this information shall submit a request under the Freedom of Information Act.

(c) Reports of adverse effects. Upon request or on its own initiative, FDA shall disclose to an individual on whom an investigational device has been used a copy of a report of adverse device effects relating to that use.

(d) Other rules. Except as otherwise provided in this section, the availability for public disclosure of data and information in an IDE file shall be handled in accordance with Sec. 814.9.

[45 FR 3751, Jan. 18, 1980, as amended at 53 FR 11253, Apr. 6, 1988; 61FR 51531, Oct. 2, 1996]

Subpart C—Responsibilities of Sponsors

Sec. 812.40 General responsibilities of sponsors.

Sponsors are responsible for selecting qualified investigators and providing them with the information they need to conduct the investigation properly, ensuring proper monitoring of the investigation, ensuring that IRB review and approval are obtained, submitting an IDE application to FDA, and ensuring that any reviewing IRB and FDA are promptly informed of significant new information about an investigation. Additional responsibilities of sponsors are described in subparts B and G.

Sec. 812.42 FDA and IRB approval.

A sponsor shall not begin an investigation or part of an investigation until an IRB and FDA have both approved the application or supplemental application relating to the investigation or part of an investigation.

[46 FR 8957, Jan. 27, 1981]

Sec. 812.43 Selecting investigators and monitors.

(a) Selecting investigators. A sponsor shall select investigators qualified by training and experience to investigate the device.

(b) Control of device. A sponsor shall ship investigational devices only to qualified investigators participating in the investigation.

(c) Obtaining agreements. A sponsor shall obtain from each participating investigator a signed agreement that includes:

(1) The investigator's curriculum vitae.

(2) Where applicable, a statement of the investigator's relevant experience, including the dates, location, extent, and type of experience.

(3) If the investigator was involved in an investigation or other research that was terminated, an explanation of the circumstances that led to termination.

(4) A statement of the investigator's commitment to:

(i) Conduct the investigation in accordance with the agreement, the investigational plan, this part and other applicable FDA regulations, and conditions of approval imposed by the reviewing IRB or FDA;

(ii) Supervise all testing of the device involving human subjects; and

(iii) Ensure that the requirements for obtaining informed consent are met.

(5) Sufficient accurate financial disclosure information to allow the sponsor to submit a complete and accurate certification or disclosure statement as required under part 54 of this chapter. The sponsor shall obtain a commitment from the clinical investigator to promptly update this information if any relevant changes occur during the course of the investigation and for 1 year following completion of the study. This information shall not be submitted in an investigational device exemption application, but shall be submitted in any marketing application involving the device.

(d) Selecting monitors. A sponsor shall select monitors qualified by training and experience to monitor the investigational study in accordance with this part and other applicable FDA regulations.

[45 FR 3751, Jan. 18, 1980, as amended at 63 FR 5253, Feb. 2, 1998] Effective Date Note: At 63 FR 5253, Feb. 2, 1998, Sec. 812.43 was amended by adding new paragraph (c)(5), effective Feb. 2, 1999.

Sec. 812.45 Informing investigators.

A sponsor shall supply all investigators participating in the investigation with copies of the investigational plan and the report of prior investigations of the device.

Sec. 812.46 Monitoring investigations.

(a) Securing compliance. A sponsor who discovers that an investigator is not complying with the signed agreement, the investigational plan, the requirements of this part or other applicable FDA regulations, or any conditions of approval imposed by the reviewing IRB or FDA shall promptly either secure compliance, or discontinue shipments of the device to the investigator and terminate the investigator's participation in the investigation. A sponsor shall also require such an investigator to dispose of or return the device, unless this action would jeopardize the rights, safety, or welfare of a subject.

(b) Unanticipated adverse device effects. (1) A sponsor shall immediately conduct an evaluation of any unanticipated adverse device effect.

(2) A sponsor who determines that an unanticipated adverse device effect presents an unreasonable risk to subjects shall terminate all investigations or parts of investigations presenting that risk as soon as possible. Termination shall occur not later than 5 working days after the sponsor makes this determination and not later than 15 working days after the sponsor first received notice of the effect.

(c) Resumption of terminated studies. If the device is a significant risk device, a sponsor may not resume a terminated investigation without IRB and FDA approval. If the device is not a significant risk device, a sponsor may not resume a terminated investigation without IRB approval and, if the investigation was terminated under paragraph (b)(2) of this section, FDA approval.

Sec. 812.47 Emergency research under Sec. 50.24 of this chapter.

(a) The sponsor shall monitor the progress of all investigations involving an exception from informed consent under Sec. 50.24 of this chapter. When the sponsor receives from the IRB information concerning the public disclosures under Sec. 50.24(a)(7)(ii) and (a)(7)(iii) of this chapter, the sponsor shall promptly submit to the IDE file and to Docket Number

95S-0158 in the Dockets Management Branch (HFA-305), Food and Drug Administration, 12420 Parklawn Dr., rm. 1-23, Rockville, MD 20857, copies of the information that was disclosed, identified by the IDE number.

(b) The sponsor also shall monitor such investigations to determine when an IRB determines that it cannot approve the research because it does not meet the criteria in the exception in Sec. 50.24(a) of this chapter or because of other relevant ethical concerns. The sponsor promptly shall provide this information in writing to FDA investigators who are asked to participate in this or a substantially equivalent clinical investigation and other IRB's that are asked to review this or a substantially equivalent investigation.

[61 FR 51531, Oct. 2, 1996]

Subpart D—IRB Review and Approval

Sec. 812.60 IRB composition, duties, and functions.

An IRB reviewing and approving investigations under this part shall comply with the requirements of part 56 in all respects, including its composition, duties, and functions.

[46 FR 8957, Jan. 27, 1981]

Sec. 812.62 IRB approval.

(a) An IRB shall review and have authority to approve, require modifications in (to secure approval), or disapprove all investigations covered by this part.

(b) If no IRB exists or if FDA finds that an IRB's review is inadequate, a sponsor may submit an application to FDA.

[46 FR 8957, Jan. 27, 1981]

Sec. 812.64 IRB's continuing review.

The IRB shall conduct its continuing review of an investigation in accordance with part 56.

[46 FR 8957, Jan. 27, 1981]

Sec. 812.66 Significant risk device determinations.

If an IRB determines that an investigation, presented for approval under Sec. 812.2(b)(1)(ii), involves a significant risk device, it shall so notify the investigator and, where appropriate, the sponsor. A sponsor may not begin the investigation except as provided in Sec. 812.30(a).

[46 FR 8957, Jan. 27, 1981]

Subpart E—Responsibilities of Investigators

Sec. 812.100 General responsibilities of investigators.

An investigator is responsible for ensuring that an investigation is conducted according to the signed agreement, the investigational plan and applicable FDA regulations, for protecting the rights, safety, and welfare of subjects under the investigator's care, and for the control of devices under investigation. An investigator also is responsible for ensuring that informed consent is obtained in accordance with part 50 of this chapter. Additional responsibilities of investigators are described in subpart G.

[45 FR 3751, Jan. 18, 1980, as amended at 46 FR 8957, Jan. 27, 1981]

Sec. 812.110 Specific responsibilities of investigators.

(a) Awaiting approval. An investigator may determine whether potential subjects would be interested in participating in an investigation, but shall not request the written informed consent of any subject to participate, and shall not allow any subject to participate before obtaining IRB and FDA approval.

(b) Compliance. An investigator shall conduct an investigation in accordance with the signed agreement with the sponsor, the investigational plan, this part and other applicable FDA regulations, and any conditions of approval imposed by an IRB or FDA.

(c) Supervising device use. An investigator shall permit an investigational device to be used only with subjects under the investigator's supervision. An investigator shall not supply an investigational device to any person not authorized under this part to receive it.

(d) Financial disclosure. A clinical investigator shall disclose to the sponsor sufficient accurate financial information to allow the applicant to submit complete and accurate certification or disclosure statements required under part 54 of this chapter. The investigator shall promptly update this information if any relevant changes occur during the course of the investigation and for 1 year following completion of the study.

(e) Disposing of device. Upon completion or termination of a clinical investigation or the investigator's part of an investigation, or at the sponsor's request, an investigator shall return to the sponsor any remaining supply of the device or otherwise dispose of the device as the sponsor directs.

[45 FR 3751, Jan. 18, 1980, as amended at 63 FR 5253, Feb. 2, 1998] Effective Date Note: At 63 FR 5253, Feb. 2, 1998, Sec. 812.110 was amended by redesignating paragraph (d) as paragraph (e) and adding new paragraph (d), effective Feb. 2, 1999.

Sec. 812.119 Disqualification of a clinical investigator.

(a) If FDA has information indicating that an investigator has repeatedly or deliberately failed to comply with the requirements of this part, part 50, or part 56 of this chapter, or has repeatedly or deliberately submitted false information either to the sponsor of the investigation or in any required report, the Center for Devices and Radiological Health will furnish the investigator written notice of the matter under complaint and offer the investigator an opportunity to explain the matter in writing, or, at the option of the investigator, in an informal conference. If an explanation is offered and accepted by the Center for Devices and Radiological Health, the disqualification process will be terminated. If an explanation is offered but not accepted by the Center for Devices and Radiological Health, the investigator will be given an opportunity for a regulatory hearing under part 16 of this chapter on the question of whether the investigator is entitled to receive investigational devices.

(b) After evaluating all available information, including any explanation presented by the investigator, if the Commissioner determines that the investigator has repeatedly or deliberately failed to comply with the requirements of this part, part 50, or part 56 of this chapter, or has deliberately or repeatedly submitted false information either to the sponsor of the investigation or in any required report, the Commissioner will notify the investigator, the sponsor of any investigation in which the investigator has been named as a participant, and the reviewing IRB that the investigator is not entitled to receive investigational devices. The notification will provide a statement of basis for such determination.

(c) Each investigational device exemption (IDE) and each cleared or approved application submitted under this part, subpart E of part 807 of this chapter, or part 814 of this chapter containing data reported by an investigator who has been determined to be ineligible to receive investigational devices will be examined to determine whether the investigator has submitted unreliable data that are essential to the continuation of the investigation or essential to the approval or clearance of any marketing application.

(d) If the Commissioner determines, after the unreliable data submitted by the investigator are eliminated from consideration, that the data remaining are inadequate to support a conclusion that it is reasonably safe to continue the investigation, the Commissioner will notify the sponsor who shall have an opportunity for a regulatory hearing under part 16 of this chapter. If a danger to the public health exists, however, the Commissioner shall terminate the IDE immediately and notify the sponsor and the reviewing IRB of the determination. In such case, the sponsor shall have an opportunity for a regulatory hearing before FDA under part 16 of this chapter on the question of whether the IDE should be reinstated.

(e) If the Commissioner determines, after the unreliable data submitted by the investigator are eliminated from consideration, that the continued clearance or approval of the marketing application for which the data were submitted cannot be justified, the

Commissioner will proceed to withdraw approval or rescind clearance of the medical device in accordance with the applicable provisions of the act.

(f) An investigator who has been determined to be ineligible to receive investigational devices may be reinstated as eligible when the Commissioner determines that the investigator has presented adequate assurances that the investigator will employ investigational devices solely in compliance with the provisions of this part and of parts 50 and 56 of this chapter.

[62 FR 12096, Mar. 14, 1997]

Subpart G—Records and Reports

Sec. 812.140 Records.

(a) Investigator records. A participating investigator shall maintain the following accurate, complete, and current records relating to the investigator's participation in an investigation:

(1) All correspondence with another investigator, an IRB, the sponsor, a monitor, or FDA, including required reports.

(2) Records of receipt, use or disposition of a device that relate to:

(i) The type and quantity of the device, the dates of its receipt, and the batch number or code mark.

(ii) The names of all persons who received, used, or disposed of each device.

(iii) Why and how many units of the device have been returned to the sponsor, repaired, or otherwise disposed of.

(3) Records of each subject's case history and exposure to the device. Case histories include the case report forms and supporting data including, for example, signed and dated consent forms and medical records including, for example, progress notes of the physician, the individual's hospital chart(s), and the nurses' notes. Such records shall include:

(i) Documents evidencing informed consent and, for any use of a device by the investigator without informed consent, any written concurrence of a licensed physician and a brief description of the circumstances justifying the failure to obtain informed consent. The case history for each individual shall document that informed consent was obtained prior to participation in the study.

(ii) All relevant observations, including records concerning adverse device effects (whether anticipated or unanticipated), information and data on the condition of each subject upon entering, and during the course of, the investigation, including information about relevant previous medical history and the results of all diagnostic tests.

(iii) A record of the exposure of each subject to the investigational device, including the date and time of each use, and any other therapy.

(4) The protocol, with documents showing the dates of and reasons for each deviation from the protocol.

(5) Any other records that FDA requires to be maintained by regulation or by specific requirement for a category of investigations or a particular investigation.

(b) Sponsor records. A sponsor shall maintain the following accurate, complete, and current records relating to an investigation:

(1) All correspondence with another sponsor, a monitor, an investigator, an IRB, or FDA, including required reports.

(2) Records of shipment and disposition. Records of shipment shall include the name and address of the consignee, type and quantity of device, date of shipment, and batch number or code mark. Records of disposition shall describe the batch number or code marks of any devices returned to the sponsor, repaired, or disposed of in other ways by the investigator or another person, and the reasons for and method of disposal.

(3) Signed investigator agreements.

(4) For each investigation subject to Sec. 812.2(b)(1) of a device other than a significant

risk device, the records described in paragraph (b)(5) of this section and the following records, consolidated in one location and available for FDA inspection and copying:

(i) The name and intended use of the device and the objectives of the investigation;

(ii) A brief explanation of why the device is not a significant risk device:

(iii) The name and address of each investigator:

(iv) The name and address of each IRB that has reviewed the investigation:

(v) A statement of the extent to which the good manufacturing practice regulation in part 820 will be followed in manufacturing the device; and

(vi) Any other information required by FDA.

(5) Records concerning adverse device effects (whether anticipated or unanticipated) and complaints and

(6) Any other records that FDA requires to be maintained by regulation or by specific requirement for a category of investigation or a particular investigation.

(c) IRB records. An IRB shall maintain records in accordance with part 56 of this chapter.

(d) Retention period. An investigator or sponsor shall maintain the records required by this subpart during the investigation and for a period of 2 years after the latter of the following two dates: The date on which the investigation is terminated or completed, or the date that the records are no longer required for purposes of supporting a premarket approval application or a notice of completion of a product development protocol.

(e) Records custody. An investigator or sponsor may withdraw from the responsibility to maintain records for the period required in paragraph (d) of this section and transfer custody of the records to any other person who will accept responsibility for them under this part, including the requirements of Sec. 812.145. Notice of a transfer shall be given to FDA not later than 10 working days after transfer occurs.

[45 FR 3751, Jan. 18, 1980, as amended at 45 FR 58843, Sept. 5, 1980; 46 FR 8957, Jan. 27, 1981; 61 FR 57280, Nov. 5, 1996]

Effective Date Note: At 63 FR 5253, Sec. 812.140 was amended by revising paragraph (b)(3), effective Feb. 2, 1999.

Sec. 812.145 Inspections.

(a) Entry and inspection. A sponsor or an investigator who has authority to grant access shall permit authorized FDA employees, at reasonable times and in a reasonable manner, to enter and inspect any establishment where devices are held (including any establishment where devices are manufactured, processed, packed, installed, used, or implanted or where records of results from use of devices are kept).

(b) Records inspection. A sponsor, IRB, or investigator, or any other person acting on behalf of such a person with respect to an investigation, shall permit authorized FDA employees, at reasonable times and in a reasonable manner, to inspect and copy all records relating to an investigation.

(c) Records identifying subjects. An investigator shall permit authorized FDA employees to inspect and copy records that identify subjects, upon notice that FDA has reason to suspect that adequate informed consent was not obtained, or that reports required to be submitted by the investigator to the sponsor or IRB have not been submitted or are incomplete, inaccurate, false, or misleading.

Sec. 812.150 Reports.

(a) Investigator reports. An investigator shall prepare and submit the following complete, accurate, and timely reports:

(1) Unanticipated adverse device effects. An investigator shall submit to the sponsor and to the reviewing IRB a report of any unanticipated adverse device effect occurring during an investigation as soon as possible, but in no event later than 10 working days after the investigator first learns of the effect.

(2) Withdrawal of IRB approval. An investigator shall report to the sponsor, within 5

working days, a withdrawal of approval by the reviewing IRB of the investigator's part of an investigation.

(3) Progress. An investigator shall submit progress reports on the investigation to the sponsor, the monitor, and the reviewing IRB at regular intervals, but in no event less often than yearly.

(4) Deviations from the investigational plan. An investigator shall notify the sponsor and the reviewing IRB (see Sec. 56.108(a) (3) and (4)) of any deviation from the investigational plan to protect the life or physical well-being of a subject in an emergency. Such notice shall be given as soon as possible, but in no event later than 5 working days after the emergency occurred. Except in such an emergency, prior approval by the sponsor is required for changes in or deviations from a plan, and if these changes or deviations may affect the scientific soundness of the plan or the rights, safety, or welfare of human subjects, FDA and IRB in accordance with Sec. 812.35(a) also is required.

(5) Informed consent. If an investigator uses a device without obtaining informed consent, the investigator shall report such use to the sponsor and the reviewing IRB within 5 working days after the use occurs.

(6) Final report. An investigator shall, within 3 months after termination or completion of the investigation or the investigator's part of the investigation, submit a final report to the sponsor and the reviewing IRB.

(7) Other. An investigator shall, upon request by a reviewing IRB or FDA, provide accurate, complete, and current information about any aspect of the investigation.

(b) Sponsor reports. A sponsor shall prepare and submit the following complete, accurate, and timely reports:

(1) Unanticipated adverse device effects. A sponsor who conducts an evaluation of an unanticipated adverse device effect under Sec. 812.46(b) shall report the results of such evaluation to FDA and to all reviewing IRB's and participating investigators within 10 working days after the sponsor first receives notice of the effect. Thereafter the sponsor shall submit such additional reports concerning the effect as FDA requests.

(2) Withdrawal of IRB approval. A sponsor shall notify FDA and all reviewing IRB's and participating investigators of any withdrawal of approval of an investigation or a part of an investigation by a reviewing IRB within 5 working days after receipt of the withdrawal of approval.

(3) Withdrawal of FDA approval. A sponsor shall notify all reviewing IRB's and participating investigators of any withdrawal of FDA approval of the investigation, and shall do so within 5 working days after receipt of notice of the withdrawal of approval.

(4) Current investigator list. A sponsor shall submit to FDA, at 6-month intervals, a current list of the names and addresses of all investigators participating in the investigation. The sponsor shall submit the first such list 6 months after FDA approval.

(5) Progress reports. At regular intervals, and at least yearly, a sponsor shall submit progress reports to all reviewing IRB's. In the case of a significant risk device, a sponsor shall also submit progress reports to FDA. A sponsor of a treatment IDE shall submit semi-annual progress reports to all reviewing IRB's and FDA in accordance with Sec. 812.36(f) and annual reports in accordance with this section.

(6) Recall and device disposition. A sponsor shall notify FDA and all reviewing IRB's of any request that an investigator return, repair, or otherwise dispose of any units of a device. Such notice shall occur within 30 working days after the request is made and shall state why the request was made.

(7) Final report. In the case of a significant risk device, the sponsor shall notify FDA within 30 working days of the completion or termination of the investigation and shall submit a final report to FDA and all reviewing the IRB's and participating investigators within 6 months after completion or termination. In the case of a device that is not a significant risk device, the sponsor shall submit a final report to all reviewing IRB's within 6 months after termination or completion.

(8) Informed consent. A sponsor shall submit to FDA a copy of any report by an inves-

tigator under paragraph (a)(5) of this section of use of a device without obtaining informed consent, within 5 working days of receipt of notice of such use.

(9) Significant risk device determinations. If an IRB determines that a device is a significant risk device, and the sponsor had proposed that the IRB consider the device not to be a significant risk device, the sponsor shall submit to FDA a report of the IRB's determination within 5 working days after the sponsor first learns of the IRB's determination.

(10) Other. A sponsor shall, upon request by a reviewing IRB or FDA, provide accurate, complete, and current information about any aspect of the investigation.

[45 FR 3751, Jan. 18, 1980, as amended at 45 FR 58843, Sept. 5, 1980; 48 FR 15622, Apr. 12, 1983; 62 FR 48948, Sept. 18, 1997]

TITLE 45 – PUBLIC WELFARE

Office for Protection from Research Risks Department of Health and Human Services

PART 46 – PROTECTION OF HUMAN SUBJECTS

Subpart A Federal Policy for the Protection of Human Subjects (Basic DHHS Policy for Protection of Human Research Subjects)

Source: 56 FR 28003, June 18, 1991.

Sec. 46.101 To what does this policy apply?

(a) Except as provided in paragraph (b) of this section, this policy applies to all research involving human subjects conducted, supported or otherwise subject to regulation by any Federal Department or Agency which takes appropriate administrative action to make the policy applicable to such research. This includes research conducted by Federal civilian employees or military personnel, except that each Department or Agency head may adopt such procedural modifications as may be appropriate from an administrative standpoint. It also includes research conducted, supported, or otherwise subject to regulation by the Federal Government outside the United States.

(1) Research that is conducted or supported by a Federal Department or Agency, whether or not it is regulated as defined in Sec. 46.102(e), must comply with all sections of this policy.

(2) Research that is neither conducted nor supported by a Federal Department or Agency but is subject to regulation as defined in Sec. 46.102(e) must be reviewed and approved, in compliance with Sec. 46.101, Sec. 46.102, and Sec. 46.107 through Sec. 46.117 of this policy, by an Institutional Review Board (IRB) that operates in accordance with the pertinent requirements of this policy.

(b) Unless otherwise required by Department or Agency heads, research activities in which the only involvement of human subjects will be in one or more of the following categories are exempt from this policy:[1]

(1) Research conducted in established or commonly accepted educational settings, involving normal educational practices, such as (i) research on regular and special education instructional strategies, or (ii) research on the effectiveness of or the comparison among instructional techniques, curricula, or classroom management methods.

(2) Research involving the use of educational tests (cognitive, diagnostic, aptitude, achievement), survey procedures, interview procedures or observation of public behavior, unless:

(i) information obtained is recorded in such a manner that human subjects can be identified, directly or through identifiers linked to the subjects; and (ii) any disclosure of the human subjects' responses outside the research could reasonably place the subjects at risk of criminal or civil liability or be damaging to the subjects' financial standing, employability, or reputation.

(3) Research involving the use of educational tests (cognitive, diagnostic, aptitude, achievement), survey procedures, interview procedures, or observation of public behavior that is not exempt under paragraph (b)(2) of this section, if:

(i) the human subjects are elected or appointed public officials or candidates for public office; or (ii) Federal statute(s) require(s) without exception that the confidentiality of the personally identifiable information will be maintained throughout the research and thereafter.

(4) Research involving the collection or study of existing data, documents, records, pathological specimens, or diagnostic specimens, if these sources are publicly available or if the information is recorded by the investigator in such a manner that subjects cannot be identified, directly or through identifiers linked to the subjects.

(5) Research and demonstration projects which are conducted by or subject to the approval of Department or Agency heads, and which are designed to study, evaluate, or otherwise examine:

(i) Public benefit or service programs; (ii) procedures for obtaining benefits or services under those programs; (iii) possible changes in or alternatives to those programs or procedures; or (iv) possible changes in methods or levels of payment for benefits or services under those programs.

(6) Taste and food quality evaluation and consumer acceptance studies, (i) if wholesome foods without additives are consumed or (ii) if a food is consumed that contains a food ingredient at or below the level and for a use found to be safe, or agricultural chemical or environmental contaminant at or below the level found to be safe, by the Food and Drug Administration or approved by the Environmental Protection Agency or the Food Safety and Inspection Service of the U.S. Department of Agriculture.

(c) Department or Agency heads retain final judgment as to whether a particular activity is covered by this policy.

(d) Department or Agency heads may require that specific research activities or classes of research activities conducted, supported, or otherwise subject to regulation by the Department or Agency but not otherwise covered by this policy, comply with some or all of the requirements of this policy.

(e) Compliance with this policy requires compliance with pertinent Federal laws or regulations which provide additional protections for human subjects.

(f) This policy does not affect any State or local laws or regulations which may otherwise be applicable and which provide additional protections for human subjects.

(g) This policy does not affect any foreign laws or regulations which may otherwise be applicable and which provide additional protections to human subjects of research.

(h) When research covered by this policy takes place in foreign countries, procedures normally followed in the foreign countries to protect human subjects may differ from those set forth in this policy. [An example is a foreign institution which complies with guidelines consistent with the World Medical Assembly Declaration (Declaration of Helsinki amended 1989) issued either by sovereign states or by an organization whose function for the protection of human research subjects is internationally recognized.] In these circumstances, if a Department or Agency head determines that the procedures prescribed by the institution afford protections that are at least equivalent to those provided in this policy, the Department or Agency head may approve the substitution of the foreign procedures in lieu of the procedural requirements provided in this policy. Except when otherwise required by statute, Executive Order, or the Department or Agency head, notices of these actions as they occur will be published in the Federal Register or will be otherwise published as provided in Department or Agency procedures.

(i) Unless otherwise required by law, Department or Agency heads may waive the applicability of some or all of the provisions of this policy to specific research activities or classes or research activities otherwise covered by this policy. Except when otherwise required by statute or Executive Order, the Department or Agencyhead shall forward advance notices of these actions to the Office for Protection from Research Risks, National Institutes of Health, Department of Health and Human Services (DHHS), and shall also publish them in the Federal Register or in such other manner as provided in Department or Agency procedures.[1]

Sec. 46.102 Definitions.

(a) Department or Agency head means the head of any Federal Department or Agency and any other officer or employee of any Department or Agency to whom authority has been delegated.

(b) Institution means any public or private entity or Agency (including Federal, State, and other agencies).

(c) Legally authorized representative means an individual or judicial or other body authorized under applicable law to consent on behalf of a prospective subject to the subject's participation in the procedure(s) involved in the research.

(d) Research means a systematic investigation, including research development, testing and evaluation, designed to develop or contribute to generalizable knowledge. Activities which meet this definition constitute research for purposes of this policy, whether or not they are conducted or supported under a program which is considered research for other purposes. For example, some demonstration and service programs may include research activities.

(e) Research subject to regulation, and similar terms are intended to encompass those research activities for which a Federal Department or Agency has specific responsibility for regulating as a research activity, (for example, Investigational New Drug requirements administered by the Food and Drug Administration). It does not include research activities which are incidentally regulated by a Federal Department or Agency solely as part of the Department's or Agency's broader responsibility to regulate certain types of activities whether research or non-research in nature (for example, Wage and Hour requirements administered by the Department of Labor).

(f) Human subject means a living individual about whom an investigator (whether professional or student) conducting research obtains

(1) data through intervention or interaction with the individual, or

(2) identifiable private information.

Intervention includes both physical procedures by which data are gathered (for example, venipuncture) and manipulations of the subject or the subject's environment that are performed for research purposes. Interaction includes communication or interpersonal contact between investigator and subject. Private information includes information about behavior that occurs in a context in which an individual can reasonably expect that no observation or recording is taking place, and information which has been provided for specific purposes by an individual and which the individual can reasonably expect will not be made public (for example, a medical record). Private information must be individually identifiable (i.e., the identity of the subject is or may readily be ascertained by the investigator or associated with the information) in order for obtaining the information to constitute research involving human subjects.

(g) IRB means an Institutional Review Board established in accord with and for the purposes expressed in this policy.

(h) IRB approval means the determination of the IRB that the research has been reviewed and may be conducted at an institution within the constraints set forth by the IRB and by other institutional and Federal requirements.

(i) Minimal risk means that the probability and magnitude of harm or discomfort anticipated in the research are not greater in and of themselves than those ordinarily encountered in daily life or during the performance of routine physical or psychological examinations or tests.

(j) Certification means the official notification by the institution to the supporting Department or Agency, in accordance with the requirements of this policy, that a research project or activity involving human subjects has been reviewed and approved by an IRB in accordance with an approved assurance.

Sec. 46.103 Assuring compliance with this policy -- research conducted or supported by any Federal Department or Agency.

(a) Each institution engaged in research which is covered by this policy and which is conducted or supported by a Federal Department or Agency shall provide written assurance satisfactory to the Department or Agency head that it will comply with the requirements set forth in this policy. In lieu of requiring submission of an assurance, individual Department or Agency heads shall accept the existence of a current assurance, appropriate for the research in question, on file with the Office for Protection from Research Risks, National Institutes Health, DHHS, and approved for Federal wide use by that office. When the existence of an DHHS-approved assurance is accepted in lieu of requiring submission of an assurance, reports (except certification) required by this policy to be made to Department and Agency heads shall also be made to the Office for Protection from Research Risks, National Institutes of Health, DHHS.

(b) Departments and agencies will conduct or support research covered by this policy only if the institution has an assurance approved as provided in this section, and only if the institution has certified to the Department or Agency head that the research has been reviewed and approved by an IRB provided for in the assurance, and will be subject to continuing review by the IRB. Assurances applicable to federally supported or conducted research shall at a minimum include:

(1) A statement of principles governing the institution in the discharge of its responsibilities for protecting the rights and welfare of human subjects of research conducted at or sponsored by the institution, regardless of whether the research is subject to Federal regulation. This may include an appropriate existing code, declaration, or statement of ethical principles, or a statement formulated by the institution itself. This requirement does not pre-empt provisions of this policy applicable to Department- or Agency-supported or regulated research and need not be applicable to any research exempted or waived under Sec. 46.101 (b) or (i).

(2) Designation of one or more IRBs established in accordance with the requirements of this policy, and for which provisions are made for meeting space and sufficient staff to support the IRB's review and recordkeeping duties.

(3) A list of IRB members identified by name; earned degrees; representative capacity; indications of experience such as board certifications, licenses, etc., sufficient to describe each member's chief anticipated contributions to IRB deliberations; and any employment or other relationship between each member and the institution; for example: full-time employee, part-time employee, member of governing panel or board, stockholder, paid or unpaid consultant. Changes in IRB membership shall be reported to the Department or Agency head, unless in accord with Sec. 46.103(a) of this policy, the existence of a DHHS-approved assurance is accepted. In this case, change in IRB membership shall be reported to the Office for Protection from Research Risks, National Institutes of Health, DHHS.

(4) Written procedures which the IRB will follow (i) for conducting its initial and continuing review of research and for reporting its findings and actions to the investigator and the institution; (ii) for determining which projects require review more often than annually and which projects need verification from sources other than the investigators that no material changes have occurred since previous IRB review; and (iii) for ensuring prompt reporting to the IRB of proposed changes in a research activity, and for ensuring that such changes in approved research, during the period for which IRB approval has already been given, may not be initiated without IRB review and approval except when necessary to eliminate apparent immediate hazards to the subject.

(5) Written procedures for ensuring prompt reporting to the IRB, appropriate institutional officials, and the Department or Agency head of (i) any unanticipated problems involving risks to subjects or others or any serious or continuing noncompliance with this policy or the requirements or determinations of the IRB; and (ii) any suspension or termi-

---

[1] Institutions with DHHS-approved assurances on file will abide by provisions of Title 45 CFR Part 46 Subparts A-D. Some of the other departments and agencies have incorporated all provisions of Title 45 CFR Part 46 into their policies and procedures as well. However, the exemptions at 45 CFR 46.101(b) do not apply to research involving prisoners, fetuses, pregnant women, or human in vitro fertilization, Subparts B and C. The exemption at 45 CFR 46.101(b)(2), for research involving survey or interview procedures or observation of public behavior, does not apply to research with children, Subpart D, except for research involving observations of public behavior when the investigator(s) do not participate in the activities being observed.

nation of IRB approval.

(c) The assurance shall be executed by an individual authorized to act for the institution and to assume on behalf of the institution the obligations imposed by this policy and shall be filed in such form and manner as the Department or Agency head prescribes.

(d) The Department or Agency head will evaluate all assurances submitted in accordance with this policy through such officers and employees of the Department or Agency and such experts or consultants engaged for this purpose as the Department or Agency head determines to be appropriate. The Department or Agency head's evaluation will take into consideration the adequacy of the proposed IRB in light of the anticipated scope of the institution's research activities and the types of subject populations likely to be involved, the appropriateness of the proposed initial and continuing review procedures in light of the probable risks, and the size and complexity of the institution.

(e) On the basis of this evaluation, the Department or Agency head may approve or disapprove the assurance, or enter into negotiations to develop an approvable one. The Department or Agency head may limit the period during which any particular approved assurance or class of approved assurances shall remain effective or otherwise condition or restrict approval.

(f) Certification is required when the research is supported by a Federal Department or Agency and not otherwise exempted or waived under Sec. 46.101 (b) or (i). An institution with an approved assurance shall certify that each application or proposal for research covered by the assurance and by Sec. 46.103 of this policy has been reviewed and approved by the IRB. Such certification must be submitted with the application or proposal or by such later date as may be prescribed by the Department or Agency to which the application or proposal is submitted. Under no condition shall research covered by Sec. 46.103 of the policy be supported prior to receipt of the certification that the research has been reviewed and approved by the IRB. Institutions without an approved assurance covering the research shall certify within 30 days after receipt of a request for such a certification from the Department or Agency, that the application or proposal has been approved by the IRB. If the certification is not submitted within these time limits, the application or proposal may be returned to the institution.

(Approved by the Office of Management and Budget under Control Number 9999-0020.)

Sec. Sec. 46.104--46.106 [Reserved]

Sec. 46.107 IRB membership.

(a) Each IRB shall have at least five members, with varying backgrounds to promote complete and adequate review of research activities commonly conducted by the institution. The IRB shall be sufficiently qualified through the experience and expertise of its members, and the diversity of the members, including consideration of race, gender, and cultural backgrounds and sensitivity to such issues as community attitudes, to promote respect for its advice and counsel in safeguarding the rights and welfare of human subjects. In addition to possessing the professional competence necessary to review specific research activities, the IRB shall be able to ascertain the acceptability of proposed research in terms of institutional commitments and regulations, applicable law, and standards of professional conduct and practice. The IRB shall therefore include persons knowledgeable in these areas. If an IRB regularly reviews research that involves a vulnerable category of subjects, such as children, prisoners, pregnant women, or handicapped or mentally disabled persons, consideration shall be given to the inclusion of one or more individuals who are knowledgeable about and experienced in working with these subjects.

(b) Every nondiscriminatory effort will be made to ensure that no IRB consists entirely of men or entirely of women, including the institution's consideration of qualified persons of both sexes, so long as no selection is made to the IRB on the basis of gender. No IRB may consist entirely of members of one profession.

(c) Each IRB shall include at least one member whose primary concerns are in scientific areas and at least one member whose primary concerns are in nonscientific areas.

(d) Each IRB shall include at least one member who is not otherwise affiliated with the institution and who is not part of the immediate family of a person who is affiliated with the institution.

(e) No IRB may have a member participate in the IRB's initial or continuing review of any project in which the member has a conflicting interest, except to provide information requested by the IRB.

(f) An IRB may, in its discretion, invite individuals with competence in special areas to assist in the review of issues which require expertise beyond or in addition to that available on the IRB. These individuals may not vote with the IRB

Sec. 46.108 IRB functions and operations.

In order to fulfill the requirements of this policy each IRB shall:

(a) Follow written procedures in the same detail as described in Sec. 46.103(b)(4) and to the extent required by Sec. 46.103(b)(5).

(b) Except when an expedited review procedure is used (see Sec. 46.110), review proposed research at convened meetings at which a majority of the members of the IRB are present, including at least one member whose primary concerns are in nonscientific areas. In order for the research to be approved, it shall receive the approval of a majority of those members present at the meeting

Sec. 46.109 IRB review of research.

(a) An IRB shall review and have authority to approve, require modifications in (to secure approval), or disapprove all research activities covered by this policy.

(b) An IRB shall require that information given to subjects as part of informed consent is in accordance with Sec. 46.116. The IRB may require that information, in addition to that specifically mentioned in Sec. 46.116, be given to the subjects when in the IRB's judgment the information would meaningfully add to the protection of the rights and welfare of subjects.

(c) An IRB shall require documentation of informed consent or may waive documentation in accordance with Sec. 46.117.

(d) An IRB shall notify investigators and the institution in writing of its decision to approve or disapprove the proposed research activity, or of modifications required to secure IRB approval of the research activity. If the IRB decides to disapprove a research activity, it shall include in its written notification a statement of the reasons for its decision and give the investigator an opportunity to respond in person or in writing.

(e) An IRB shall conduct continuing review of research covered by this policy at intervals appropriate to the degree of risk, but not less than once per year, and shall have authority to observe or have a third party observe the consent process and the research.

(Approved by the Office of Management and Budget under Control Number 9999-0020.)

Sec. 46.110 Expedited review procedures for certain kinds of research involving no more than minimal risk, and for minor changes in approved research.

(a) The Secretary, HHS, has established, and published as a Notice in the Federal Register, a list of categories of research that may be reviewed by the IRB through an expedited review procedure. The list will be amended, as appropriate, after consultation with other departments and agencies, through periodic republication by the Secretary, HHS, in the Federal Register. A copy of the list is available from the Office for Protection from Research Risks, National Institutes of Health, DHHS, Bethesda, Maryland 20892.

(b) An IRB may use the expedited review procedure to review either or both of the following:

(1) some or all of the research appearing on the list and found by the reviewer(s) to involve no more than minimal risk,

(2) minor changes in previously approved research during the period (of one year or less) for which approval is authorized.

Under an expedited review procedure, the review may be carried out by the IRB chairperson or by one or more experienced reviewers designated by the chairperson from among members of the IRB. In reviewing the research, the reviewers may exercise all of the authorities of the IRB except that the reviewers may not disapprove the research. A research activity may be disapproved only after review in accordance with the non-expedited procedure set forth in Sec. 46.108(b).

(c) Each IRB which uses an expedited review procedure shall adopt a method for keeping all members advised of research proposals which have been approved under the procedure.

(d) The Department or Agency head may restrict, suspend, terminate, or choose not to authorize an institution's or IRB's use of the expedited review procedure.

Sec. 46.111 Criteria for IRB approval of research.

(a) In order to approve research covered by this policy the IRB shall determine that all of the following requirements are satisfied:

(1) Risks to subjects are minimized: (i) by using procedures which are consistent with sound research design and which do not unnecessarily expose subjects to risk, and (ii) whenever appropriate, by using procedures already being performed on the subjects for diagnostic or treatment purposes.

(2) Risks to subjects are reasonable in relation to anticipated benefits, if any, to subjects, and the importance of the knowledge that may reasonably be expected to result. In evaluating risks and benefits, the IRB should consider only those risks and benefits that may result from the research (as distinguished from risks and benefits of therapies subjects would receive even if not participating in the research). The IRB should not consider possible long-range effects of applying knowledge gained in the research (for example, the possible effects of the research on public policy) as among those research risks that fall within the purview of its responsibility.

(3) Selection of subjects is equitable. In making this assessment the IRB should take into account the purposes of the research and the setting in which the research will be conducted and should be particularly cognizant of the special problems of research involving vulnerable populations, such as children, prisoners, pregnant women, mentally disable persons, or economically or educationally disadvantaged persons.

(4) Informed consent will be sought from each prospective subject or the subject's legally authorized representative, in accordance with, and to the extent required by Sec. 46.116.

(5) Informed consent will be appropriately documented, in accordance with, and to the extent required by Sec. 46.117.

(6) When appropriate, the research plan makes adequate provision for monitoring the data collected to ensure the safety of subjects.

(7) When appropriate, there are adequate provisions to protect the privacy of subjects and to maintain the confidentiality of data.

(b) When some or all of the subjects are likely to be vulnerable to coercion or undue influence, such as children, prisoners, pregnant women, mentally disabled persons, or economically or educationally disadvantaged persons, additional safeguards have been included in the study to protect the rights and welfare of these subjects.

Sec. 46.112 Review by institution.

Research covered by this policy that has been approved by an IRB may be subject to further appropriate review and approval or disapproval by officials of the institution. However, those officials may not approve the research if it has not been approved by an IRB.

Sec. 46.113 Suspension or termination of IRB approval of research.

An IRB shall have authority to suspend or terminate approval of research that is not being conducted in accordance with the IRB's requirements or that has been associated with unexpected serious harm to subjects. Any suspension or termination or approval shall include a statement of the reasons for the IRB's action and shall be reported promptly to the investigator, appropriate institutional officials, and the Department or Agency head.

(Approved by the Office of Management and Budget under Control Number 9999-0020.)

Sec. 46.114 Cooperative research.

Cooperative research projects are those projects covered by this policy which involve more than one institution. In the conduct of cooperative research projects, each institution is responsible for safeguarding the rights and welfare of human subjects and for complying with this policy. With the approval of the Department or Agency head, an institution participating in a cooperative project may enter into a joint review arrangement, rely upon the review of another qualified IRB, or make similar arrangements for avoiding duplication of effort.

Sec. 46.115 IRB records.

(a) An institution, or when appropriate an IRB, shall prepare and maintain adequate documentation of IRB activities, including the following:

(1) Copies of all research proposals reviewed, scientific evaluations, if any, that accompany the proposals, approved sample consent documents, progress reports submitted by investigators, and reports of injuries to subjects.

(2) Minutes of IRB meetings which shall be in sufficient detail to show attendance at the meetings; actions taken by the IRB; the vote on these actions including the number of members voting for, against, and abstaining; the basis for requiring changes in or disapproving research; and a written summary of the discussion of controverted issues and their resolution.

(3) Records of continuing review activities.

(4) Copies of all correspondence between the IRB and the investigators.

(5) A list of IRB members in the same detail as described in Sec. 46.103(b)(3).

(6) Written procedures for the IRB in the same detail as described in Sec. 46.103(b)(4) and Sec. 46.103(b)(5).

(7) Statements of significant new findings provided to subjects, as required by Sec. 46.116(b)(5).

(b) The records required by this policy shall be retained for at least 3 years, and records relating to research which is conducted shall be retained for at least 3 years after completion of the research. All records shall be accessible for inspection and copying by authorized representatives of the Department or Agency at reasonable times and in a reasonable manner.

(Approved by the Office of Management and Budget under Control Number 9999-0020.)

Sec. 46.116 General requirements for informed consent.

Except as provided elsewhere in this policy, no investigator may involve a human being as a subject in research covered by this policy unless the investigator has obtained the legally effective informed consent of the subject or the subject's legally authorized representative. An investigator shall seek such consent only under circumstances that provide the prospective subject or the representative sufficient opportunity to consider whether or not to participate and that minimize the possibility of coercion or undue influence. The information that is given to the subject or the representative shall be in language understandable to the subject or the representative. No informed consent, whether oral or written, may include any exculpatory language through which the subject or the representative is made to waive or appear to waive any of the subject's legal rights, or releases or appears to release the investigator, the sponsor, the institution or its agents from liability for negligence.

(a) Basic elements of informed consent. Except as provided in paragraph (c) or (d) of this section, in seeking informed consent the following information shall be provided to each subject:

(1) a statement that the study involves research, an explanation of the purposes of the research and the expected duration of the subject's participation, a description of the proce-

dures to be followed, and identification of any procedures which are experimental;

(2) a description of any reasonably foreseeable risks or discomforts to the subject;

(3) a description of any benefits to the subject or to others which may reasonably be expected from the research;

(4) a disclosure of appropriate alternative procedures or courses of treatment, if any, that might be advantageous to the subject;

(5) a statement describing the extent, if any, to which confidentiality of records identifying the subject will be maintained;

(6) for research involving more than minimal risk, an explanation as to whether any compensation and an explanation as to whether any medical treatments are available if injury occurs and, if so, what they consist of, or where further information may be obtained;

(7) an explanation of whom to contact for answers to pertinent questions about the research and research subjects' rights, and whom to contact in the event of a research-related injury to the subject; and

(8) a statement that participation is voluntary, refusal to participate will involve no penalty or loss of benefits to which the subject is otherwise entitled, and the subject may discontinue participation at any time without penalty or loss of benefits to which the subject is otherwise entitled.

(b) additional elements of informed consent. When appropriate, one or more of the following elements of information shall also be provided to each subject:

(1) a statement that the particular treatment or procedure may involve risks to the subject (or to the embryo or fetus, if the subject is or may become pregnant) which are currently unforeseeable;

(2) anticipated circumstances under which the subject's participation may be terminated by the investigator without regard to the subject's consent;

(3) any additional costs to the subject that may result from participation in the research;

(4) the consequences of a subject's decision to withdraw from the research and procedures for orderly termination of participation by the subject;

(5) A statement that significant new findings developed during the course of the research which may relate to the subject's willingness to continue participation will be provided to the subject; and

(6) the approximate number of subjects involved in the study.

(c) An IRB may approve a consent procedure which does not include, or which alters, some or all of the elements of informed consent set forth above, or waive the requirement to obtain informed consent provided the IRB finds and documents that:

(1) the research or demonstration project is to be conducted by or subject to the approval of state or local government officials and is designed to study, evaluate, or otherwise examine: (i) public benefit or service programs;

(ii) procedures for obtaining benefits or services under those programs; (iii) possible changes in or alternatives to those programs or procedures; or (iv) possible changes in methods or levels of payment for benefits or services under those programs; and

(2) the research could not practicably be carried out without the waiver or alteration.

(d) An IRB may approve a consent procedure which does not include, or which alters, some or all of the elements of informed consent set forth in this section, or waive the requirements to obtain informed consent provided the IRB finds and documents that:

(1) the research involves no more than minimal risk to the subjects;

(2) the waiver or alteration will not adversely affect the rights and welfare of the subjects;

(3) the research could not practicably be carried out without the waiver or alteration; and

(4) whenever appropriate, the subjects will be provided with additional pertinent information after participation.

(e) The informed consent requirements in this policy are not intended to preempt any applicable Federal, State, or local laws which require additional information to be disclosed in order for informed consent to be legally effective.

(f) Nothing in this policy is intended to limit the authority of a physician to provide emergency medical care, to the extent the physician is permitted to do so under applicable Federal, State, or local law.

(Approved by the Office of Management and Budget under Control Number 9999-0020.)

Sec. 46.117 Documentation of informed consent.

(a) Except as provided in paragraph (c) of this section, informed consent shall be documented by the use of a written consent form approved by the IRB and signed by the subject or the subject's legally authorized representative. A copy shall be given to the person signing the form.

(b) Except as provided in paragraph (c) of this section, the consent form may be either of the following:

(1) A written consent document that embodies the elements of informed consent required by Sec. 46.116. This form may be read to the subject or the subject's legally authorized representative, but in any event, the investigator shall give either the subject or the representative adequate opportunity to read it before it is signed; or

(2) A short form written consent document stating that the elements of informed consent required by Sec. 46.116 have been presented orally to the subject or the subject's legally authorized representative. When this method is used, there shall be a witness to the oral presentation. Also, the IRB shall approve a written summary of what is to be said to the subject or the representative. Only the short form itself is to be signed by the subject or the representative.

However, the witness shall sign both the short form and a copy of the summary, and the person actually obtaining consent shall sign a copy of the summary. A copy of the summary shall be given to the subject or the representative, in addition to a copy of the short form.

(c) An IRB may waive the requirement for the investigator to obtain a signed consent form for some or all subjects if it finds either:

(1) That the only record linking the subject and the research would be the consent document and the principal risk would be potential harm resulting from a breach of confidentiality. Each subject will be asked whether the subject wants documentation linking the subject with the research, and the subject's wishes will govern; or

(2) That the research presents no more than minimal risk of harm to subjects and involves no procedures for which written consent is normally required outside of the research context.

In cases in which the documentation requirement is waived, the IRB may require the investigator to provide subjects with a written statement regarding the research.

(Approved by the Office of Management and Budget under Control Number 9999-0020.)

Sec. 46.118 Applications and proposals lacking definite plans for involvement of human subjects.

Certain types of applications for grants, cooperative agreements, or contracts are submitted to departments or agencies with the knowledge that subjects may be involved within the period of support, but definite plans would not normally be set forth in the application or proposal. These include activities such as institutional type grants when selection of specific projects is the institution's responsibility; research training grants in which the activities involving subjects remain to be selected; and projects in which human subjects' involvement will depend upon completion of instruments, prior animal studies, or purification of compounds. These applications need not be reviewed by an IRB before an award may be made. However, except for research exempted or waived under Sec. 46.101 (b) or (i), no human subjects may be involved in any project supported by these awards until the project has been reviewed and approved by the IRB, as provided in this policy, and certification submitted, by the institution, to the Department or Agency.

Sec. 46.119 Research undertaken without the intention of involving human subjects.

In the event research is undertaken without the intention of involving human subjects, but it is later proposed to involve human subjects in the research, the research shall first be reviewed and approved by an IRB, as provided in this policy, a certification submitted, by the institution, to the Department or Agency, and final approval given to the proposed change by the Department or Agency.

Sec. 46.120 Evaluation and disposition of applications and proposals for research to be conducted or supported by a Federal Department or Agency.

(a) The Department or Agency head will evaluate all applications and proposals involving human subjects submitted to the Department or Agency through such officers and employees of the Department or Agency and such experts and consultants as the Department or Agency head determines to be appropriate. This evaluation will take into consideration the risks to the subjects, the adequacy of protection against these risks, the potential benefits of the research to the subjects and others, and the importance of the knowledge gained or to be gained.

(b) On the basis of this evaluation, the Department or Agency head may approve or disapprove the application or proposal, or enter into negotiations to develop an approvable one.

Sec. 46.121 [Reserved]

Sec. 46.122 Use of Federal funds.

Federal funds administered by a Department or Agency may not be expended for research involving human subjects unless the requirements of this policy have been satisfied.

Sec. 46.123 Early termination of research support: Evaluation of applications and proposals.

(a) The Department or Agency head may require that Department or Agency support for any project be terminated or suspended in the manner prescribed in applicable program requirements, when the Department or Agency head finds an institution has materially failed to comply with the terms of this policy.

(b) In making decisions about supporting or approving applications or proposals covered by this policy the Department or Agency head may take into account, in addition to all other eligibility requirements and program criteria, factors such as whether the applicant has been subject to a termination or suspension under paragraph (a) of this section and whether the applicant or the person or persons who would direct or has/have directed the scientific and technical aspects of an activity has/have, in the judgment of the Department or Agency head, materially failed to discharge responsibility for the protection of the rights and welfare of human subjects (whether or not the research was subject to Federal regulation).

Sec. 46.124 Conditions.

With respect to any research project or any class of research projects the Department or Agency head may impose additional conditions prior to or at the time of approval when in the judgment of the Department or Agency head additional conditions are necessary for the protection of human subjects.

Subpart B

Additional DHHS Protections Pertaining to Research, Development, and Related Activities Involving Fetuses, Pregnant Women, and Human In Vitro Fertilization

Source: 40 FR 33528, Aug. 8, 1975; 43 FR 1758, January 11, 1978; 43 FR 51559, November 3, 1978.

Sec. 46.201 Applicability.

(a) The regulations in this subpart are applicable to all Department of Health and Human Services grants and contracts supporting research, development, and related activities involving: (1) the fetus, (2) pregnant women, and (3) human in vitro fertilization.

(b) Nothing in this subpart shall be construed as indicating that compliance with the procedures set forth herein will in any way render inapplicable pertinent State or local laws bearing upon activities covered by this subpart.

(c) The requirements of this subpart are in addition to those imposed under the other subparts of this part.

Sec. 46.202 Purpose.

It is the purpose of this subpart to provide additional safeguards in reviewing activities to which this subpart is applicable to assure that they conform to appropriate ethical standards and relate to important societal needs.

Sec. 46.203 Definitions.

As used in this subpart:

(a) "Secretary" means the Secretary of Health and Human Services and any other officer or employee of the Department of Health and Human Services (DHHS) to whom authority has been delegated.

(b) "Pregnancy" encompasses the period of time from confirmation of implantation (through any of the presumptive signs of pregnancy, such as missed menses, or by a medically acceptable pregnancy test), until expulsion or extraction of the fetus.

(c) "Fetus" means the product of conception from the time of implantation (as evidenced by any of the presumptive signs of pregnancy, such as missed menses, or a medically acceptable pregnancy test), until a determination is made, following expulsion or extraction of the fetus, that it is viable.

(d) "Viable" as it pertains to the fetus means being able, after either spontaneous or induced delivery, to survive (given the benefit of available medical therapy) to the point of independently maintaining heart beat and respiration. The Secretary may from time to time, taking into account medical advances, publish in the Federal Register guidelines to assist in determining whether a fetus is viable for purposes of this subpart. If a fetus is viable after delivery, it is a premature infant.

(e) "Nonviable fetus" means a fetus ex utero which, although living, is not viable.

(f) "Dead fetus" means a fetus ex utero which exhibits neither heartbeat, spontaneous respiratory activity, spontaneous movement of voluntary muscles, nor pulsation of the umbilical cord (if still attached).

(g) "In vitro fertilization" means any fertilization of human ova which occurs outside the body of a female, either through admixture of donor human sperm and ova or by any other means.

Sec. 46.204 Ethical Advisory Boards.

(a) One or more Ethical Advisory Boards shall be established by the Secretary. Members of these Board(s) shall be so selected that the Board(s) will be competent to deal with medical, legal, social, ethical, and related issues and may include, for example, research scientists, physicians, psychologists, sociologists, educators, lawyers, and ethicists, as well as representatives of the general public. No Board member may be a regular, full-time employee of the Department of Health and Human Services.

(b) At the request of the Secretary, the Ethical Advisory Board shall render advice consistent with the policies and requirements of this part as to ethical issues, involving activities covered by this subpart, raised by individual applications or proposals. In addition, upon request by the Secretary, the Board shall render advice as to classes of applications or proposals and general policies, guidelines, and procedures.

(c) A Board may establish, with the approval of the Secretary, classes of applications or proposals which: (1) must be submitted to the Board, or (2) need not be submitted to the Board. Where the Board so establishes a class ofapplications or proposals which must be submitted, no application or proposal within the class may be funded by the Department or any component thereof until the application or proposal has been reviewed by the Board and the Board has rendered advice as to its acceptability from an ethical standpoint.

(d) [Nullified under Public Law 103-43, June 10, 1993]

Sec. 46.205 Additional duties of the Institutional Review Boards in connection with activities involving fetuses, pregnant women, or human in vitro fertilization.

(a) In addition to the responsibilities prescribed for Institutional Review Boards under Subpart A of this part, the applicant's or offeror's Board shall, with respect to activities covered by this subpart, carry out the following additional duties:

(1) determine that all aspects of the activity meet the requirements of this subpart;

(2) determine that adequate consideration has been given to the manner in which potential subjects will be selected, and adequate provision has been made by the applicant or offeror for monitoring the actual informed consent process (e.g., through such mechanisms, when appropriate, as participation by the Institutional Review Board or subject advocates in: (i) overseeing the actual process by which individual consents required by this subpart are secured either by approving induction of each individual into the activity or verifying, perhaps through sampling, that approved procedures for induction of individuals into the activity are being followed, and (ii) monitoring the progress of the activity and intervening as necessary through such steps as visits to the activity site and continuing evaluation to determine if any unanticipated risks have arisen);

(3) carry out such other responsibilities as may be assigned by the Secretary.

(b) No award may be issued until the applicant or offeror has certified to the Secretary that the Institutional Review Board has made the determinations required under paragraph (a) of this section and the Secretary has approved these determinations, as provided in Sec. 46.120 of Subpart A of this part.

(c) Applicants or offerors seeking support for activities covered by this subpart must provide for the designation of an Institutional Review Board, subject to approval by the Secretary, where no such Board has been established under Subpart A of this part.

Sec. 46.206 General limitations.

(a) No activity to which this subpart is applicable may be undertaken unless:

(1) appropriate studies on animals and nonpregnant individuals have been completed;

(2) except where the purpose of the activity is to meet the health needs of the mother or the particular fetus, the risk to the fetus is minimal and, in all cases, is the least possible risk for achieving the objectives of the activity;

(3) individuals engaged in the activity will have no part in: (i) any decisions as to the timing, method, and procedures used to terminate the pregnancy, and (ii) determining the viability of the fetus at the termination of the pregnancy; and

(4) no procedural changes which may cause greater than minimal risk to the fetus or the pregnant woman will be introduced into the procedure for terminating the pregnancy solely in the interest of the activity.

(b) No inducements, monetary or otherwise, may be offered to terminate pregnancy for purposes of the activity.

Source: 40 FR 33528, Aug. 8, 1975, as amended at 40 FR 51638, Nov. 6, 1975.

Sec. 46.207 Activities directed toward pregnant women as subjects.

(a) No pregnant woman may be involved as a subject in an activity covered by this subpart unless: (1) the purpose of the activity is to meet the health needs of the mother and the fetus will be placed at risk only to the minimum extent necessary to meet such needs, or (2) the risk to the fetus is minimal.

(b) An activity permitted under paragraph (a) of this section may be conducted only if the mother and father are legally competent and have given their informed consent after having been fully informed regarding possible impact on the fetus, except that the father's informed consent need not be secured if: (1) the purpose of the activity is to meet the health needs of the mother; (2) his identity or whereabouts cannot reasonably be ascertained; (3) he is not reasonably available; or (4) the pregnancy resulted from rape.

Sec. 46.208 Activities directed toward fetuses in utero as subjects.

(a) No fetus in utero may be involved as a subject in any activity covered by this subpart unless: (1) the purpose of the activity is to meet the health needs of the particular fetus and the fetus will be placed at risk only to the minimum extent necessary to meet such needs, or (2) the risk to the fetus imposed by the research is minimal and the purpose of the activity is the development of important biomedical knowledge which cannot be obtained by other means.

(b) An activity permitted under paragraph (a) of this section may be conducted only if the mother and father are legally competent and have given their informed consent, except that the father's consent need not be secured if: (1) his identity or whereabouts cannot reasonably be ascertained, (2) he is not reasonably available, or (3) the pregnancy resulted from rape.

Sec. 46.209 Activities directed toward fetuses ex utero, including nonviable fetuses, as subjects.

(a) Until it has been ascertained whether or not a fetus ex utero is viable, a fetus ex utero may not be involved as a subject in an activity covered by this subpart unless:

(1) there will be no added risk to the fetus resulting from the activity, and the purpose of the activity is the development of important biomedical knowledge which cannot be obtained by other means, or

(2) the purpose of the activity is to enhance the possibility of survival of the particular fetus to the point of viability.

(b) No nonviable fetus may be involved as a subject in an activity covered by this subpart unless:

(1) vital functions of the fetus will not be artificially maintained,

(2) experimental activities which of themselves would terminate the heartbeat or respiration of the fetus will not be employed, and

(3) the purpose of the activity is the development of important biomedical knowledge which cannot be obtained by other means.

(c) In the event the fetus ex utero is found to be viable, it may be included as a subject in the activity only to the extent permitted by and in accordance with the requirements of other subparts of this part.

(d) An activity permitted under paragraph (a) or (b) of this section may be conducted only if the mother and father are legally competent and have given their informed consent, except that the father's informed consent need not be secured if: (1) his identity or whereabouts cannot reasonably be ascertained, (2) he is not reasonably available, or (3) the pregnancy resulted from rape.

Sec. 46.210 Activities involving the dead fetus, fetal material, or the placenta.

Activities involving the dead fetus, mascerated fetal material, or cells, tissue, or organs excised from a dead fetus shall be conducted only in accordance with any applicable State or local laws regarding such activities.

Sec. 46.211 Modification or waiver of specific requirements.

Upon the request of an applicant or offeror (with the approval of its Institutional Review Board), the Secretary may modify or waive specific requirements of this subpart, with the approval of the Ethical Advisory Board after such opportunity for public comment as the Ethical Advisory Board considers appropriate in the particular instance. In making such decisions, the Secretary will consider whether the risks to the subject are so outweighed

208

by the sum of the benefit to the subject and the importance of the knowledge to be gained as to warrant such modification or waiver and that such benefits cannot be gained except through a modification or waiver. Any such modifications or waivers will be published as notices in the Federal Register.

Subpart C

Additional DHHS Protections Pertaining to Biomedical and Behavioral Research Involving Prisoners as Subjects

Source: 43 FR 53655, Nov. 16, 1978.

Sec. 46.301 Applicability.

(a) The regulations in this subpart are applicable to all biomedical and behavioral research conducted or supported by the Department of Health and Human Services involving prisoners as subjects.

(b) Nothing in this subpart shall be construed as indicating that compliance with the procedures set forth herein will authorize research involving prisoners as subjects, to the extent such research is limited or barred by applicable State or local law.

(c) The requirements of this subpart are in addition to those imposed under the other subparts of this part.

Sec. 46.302 Purpose.

Inasmuch as prisoners may be under constraints because of their incarceration which could affect their ability to make a truly voluntary and uncoerced decision whether or not to participate as subjects in research, it is the purpose of this subpart to provide additional safeguards for the protection of prisoners involved in activities to which this subpart is applicable.

Sec. 46.303 Definitions.

As used in this subpart:

(a) "Secretary" means the Secretary of Health and Human Services and any other officer or employee of the Department of Health and Human Services to whom authority has been delegated.

(b) "DHHS" means the Department of Health and Human Services.

(c) "Prisoner" means any individual involuntarily confined or detained in a penal institution. The term is intended to encompass individuals sentenced to such an institution under a criminal or civil statute, individuals detained in other facilities by virtue of statutes or commitment procedures which provide alternatives to criminal prosecution or incarceration in a penal institution, and individuals detained pending arraignment, trial, or sentencing.

(d) "Minimal risk" is the probability and magnitude of physical or psychological harm that is normally encountered in the daily lives, or in the routine medical, dental, or psychological examination of healthy persons.

Sec. 46.304 Composition of Institutional Review Boards where prisoners are involved.

In addition to satisfying the requirements in Sec. 46.107 of this part, an Institutional Review Board, carrying out responsibilities under this part with respect to research covered by this subpart, shall also meet the following specific requirements:

(a) A majority of the Board (exclusive of prisoner members) shall have no association with the prison(s) involved, apart from their membership on the Board.

(b) At least one member of the Board shall be a prisoner, or a prisoner representative with appropriate background and experience to serve in that capacity, except that where a particular research project is reviewed by more than one Board only one Board need satisfy this requirement.

Sec. 46.305 Additional duties of the Institutional Review Boards where prisoners are involved.

(a) In addition to all other responsibilities prescribed for Institutional Review Boards under this part, the Board shall review research covered by this subpart and approve such research only if it finds that:

(1) the research under review represents one of the categories of research permissible under Sec. 46.306(a)(2);

(2) any possible advantages accruing to the prisoner through his or her participation in the research, when compared to the general living conditions, medical care, quality of food, amenities and opportunity for earnings in the prison, are not of such a magnitude that his or her ability to weigh the risks of the research against the value of such advantages in the limited choice environment of the prison is impaired;

(3) the risks involved in the research are commensurate with risks that would be accepted by nonprisoner volunteers;

(4) procedures for the selection of subjects within the prison are fair to all prisoners and immune from arbitrary intervention by prison authorities or prisoners. Unless the principal investigator provides to the Board justification in writing for following some other procedures, control subjects must be selected randomly from the group of available prisoners who meet the characteristics needed for that particular research project;

(5) the information is presented in language which is understandable to the subject population;

(6) adequate assurance exists that parole boards will not take into account a prisoner's participation in the research in making decisions regarding parole, and each prisoner is clearly informed in advance that participation in the research will have no effect on his or her parole; and

(7) where the Board finds there may be a need for follow-up examination or care of participants after the end of their participation, adequate provision has been made for such examination or care, taking into account the varying lengths of individual prisoners' sentences, and for informing participants of this fact.

(b) The Board shall carry out such other duties as may be assigned by the Secretary.

(c) The institution shall certify to the Secretary, in such form and manner as the Secretary may require, that the duties of the Board under this section have been fulfilled.

Sec. 46.306 Permitted research involving prisoners.

(a) Biomedical or behavioral research conducted or supported by DHHS may involve prisoners as subjects only if:

(1) the institution responsible for the conduct of the research has certified to the Secretary that the Institutional Review Board has approved the research under Sec. 46.305 of this subpart; and

(2) in the judgment of the Secretary the proposed research involves solely the following:

(A) study of the possible causes, effects, and processes of incarceration, and of criminal behavior, provided that the study presents no more than minimal risk and no more than inconvenience to the subjects;

(B) study of prisons as institutional structures or of prisoners as incarcerated persons, provided that the study presents no more than minimal risk and no more than inconvenience to the subjects;

(C) research on conditions particularly affecting prisoners as a class (for example, vaccine trials and other research on hepatitis which is much more prevalent in prisons than elsewhere; and research on social and psychological problems such as alcoholism, drug addiction, and sexual assaults) provided that the study may proceed only after the Secretary has consulted with appropriate experts including experts in penology, medicine, and ethics, and published notice, in the Federal Register, of his intent to approve such research; or

(D) research on practices, both innovative and accepted, which have the intent and reasonable probability of improving the health or well-being of the subject. In cases in which those studies require the assignment of prisoners in a manner consistent with protocols approved by the IRB to control groups which may not benefit from the research, the study may proceed only after the Secretary has consulted with appropriate experts, including experts in penology, medicine, and ethics, and published notice, in the Federal Register, of the intent to approve such research.

(b) Except as provided in paragraph (a) of this section, biomedical or behavioral research conducted or supported by DHHS shall not involve prisoners as subjects.

Subpart D

Additional DHHS Protections for Children Involved as Subjects in Research
Source: 48 FR 9818, March 8, 1983; 56 FR 28032, June 18, 1991.

Sec. 46.401 To what do these regulations apply?

(a) This subpart applies to all research involving children as subjects, conducted or supported by the Department of Health and Human Services.

(1) This includes research conducted by Department employees, except that each head of an Operating Division of the Department may adopt such nonsubstantive, procedural modifications as may be appropriate from an administrative standpoint.

(2) It also includes research conducted or supported by the Department of Health and Human Services outside the United States, but in appropriate circumstances, the Secretary may, under paragraph (i) of Sec. 46.101 of Subpart A, waive the applicability of some or all of the requirements of these regulations for research of this type.

(b) Exemptions at Sec. 46.101(b)(1) and (b)(3) through (b)(6) are applicable to this subpart. The exemption at Sec. 46.101(b)(2) regarding educational tests is also applicable to this subpart. However, the exemption at Sec. 46.101(b)(2) for research involving survey or interview procedures or observations of public behavior does not apply to research covered by this subpart, except for research involving observation of public behavior when the investigator(s) do not participate in the activities being observed.

(c) The exceptions, additions, and provisions for waiver as they appear in paragraphs (c) through (i) of Sec. 46.101 of Subpart A are applicable to this subpart.

Sec. 46.402 Definitions.

The definitions in Sec. 46.102 of Subpart A shall be applicable to this subpart as well. In addition, as used in this subpart:

(a) "Children" are persons who have not attained the legal age for consent to treatments or procedures involved in the research, under the applicable law of the jurisdiction in which the research will be conducted.

(b) "Assent" means a child's affirmative agreement to participate in research. Mere failure to object should not, absent affirmative agreement, be construed as assent.

(c) "Permission" means the agreement of parent(s) or guardian to the participation of their child or ward in research.

(d) "Parent" means a child's biological or adoptive parent.

(e) "Guardian" means an individual who is authorized under applicable State or local law to consent on behalf of a child to general medical care.

Sec. 46.403 IRB duties.

In addition to other responsibilities assigned to IRBs under this part, each IRB shall review research covered by this subpart and approve only research which satisfies the conditions of all applicable sections of this subpart.

Sec. 46.404 Research not involving greater than minimal risk.

DHHS will conduct or fund research in which the IRB finds that no greater than minimal risk to children is presented, only if the IRB finds that adequate provisions are made for soliciting the assent of the children and the permission of their parents or guardians, as set forth in Sec. 46.408.

Sec. 46.405 Research involving greater than minimal risk but presenting the prospect of direct benefit to the individual subjects.

DHHS will conduct or fund research in which the IRB finds that more than minimal risk to children is presented by an intervention or procedure that holds out the prospect of direct benefit for the individual subject, or by a monitoring procedure that is likely to contribute to the subject's well-being, only if the IRB finds that:

(a) the risk is justified by the anticipated benefit to the subjects;

(b) the relation of the anticipated benefit to the risk is at least as favorable to the subjects as that presented by available alternative approaches; and

(c) adequate provisions are made for soliciting the assent of the children and permission of their parents or guardians, as set forth in Sec. 46.408.

Sec. 46.406 Research involving greater than minimal risk and no prospect of direct benefit to individual subjects, but likely to yield generalizable knowledge about the subject's disorder or condition.

DHHS will conduct or fund research in which the IRB finds that more than minimal risk to children is presented by an intervention or procedure that does not hold out the prospect of direct benefit for the individual subject, or by a monitoring procedure which is not likely to contribute to the well-being of the subject, only if the IRB finds that:

(a) the risk represents a minor increase over minimal risk;

(b) the intervention or procedure presents experiences to subjects that are reasonably commensurate with those inherent in their actual or expected medical, dental, psychological, social, or educational situations;

(c) the intervention or procedure is likely to yield generalizable knowledge about the subjects' disorder or condition which is of vital importance for the understanding or amelioration of the subjects' disorder or condition; and

(d) adequate provisions are made for soliciting assent of the children and permission of their parents or guardians, as set forth in Sec. 46.408.

Sec. 46.407 Research not otherwise approvable which presents an opportunity to understand, prevent, or alleviate a serious problem affecting the health or welfare of children.

DHHS will conduct or fund research that the IRB does not believe meets the requirements of Sec. 46.404, Sec. 46.405, or Sec. 46.406 only if:

(a) the IRB finds that the research presents a reasonable opportunity to further the understanding, prevention, or alleviation of a serious problem affecting the health or welfare of children; and

(b) the Secretary, after consultation with a panel of experts in pertinent disciplines (for example: science, medicine, education, ethics, law) and following opportunity for public review and comment, has determined either:

(1) that the research in fact satisfies the conditions of Sec. 46.404, Sec. 46.405, or Sec. 46.406, as applicable, or (2) the following:

(i) the research presents a reasonable opportunity to further the understanding, prevention, or alleviation of a serious problem affecting the health or welfare of children;

(ii) the research will be conducted in accordance with sound ethical principles;

(iii) adequate provisions are made for soliciting the assent of children and the permission of their parents or guardians, as set forth in Sec. 46.408.

Sec. 46.408 Requirements for permission by parents or guardians and for assent by children.

(a) In addition to the determinations required under other applicable sections of this subpart, the IRB shall determine that adequate provisions are made for soliciting the assent of the children, when in the judgment of the IRB the children are capable of providing assent. In determining whether children are capable of assenting, the IRB shall take into account the ages, maturity, and psychological state of the children involved. This judgment may be made for all children to be involved in research under a particular protocol, or for each child, as the IRB deems appropriate. If the IRB determines that the capability of some or all of the children is so limited that they cannot reasonably be consulted or that the intervention or procedure involved in the research holds out a prospect of direct benefit that is important to the health or well-being of the children and is available only in the context of the research, the assent of the children is not a necessary condition for proceeding with the research. Even where the IRB determines that the subjects are capable of assenting, the IRB may still waive the assent requirement under circumstances in which consent may be waived in accord with Sec. 46.116 of Subpart A.

(b) In addition to the determinations required under other applicable sections of this subpart, the IRB shall determine, in accordance with and to the extent that consent is required by Sec. 46.116 of Subpart A, that adequate provisions are made for soliciting the permission of each child's parents or guardian. Where parental permission is to be obtained, the IRB may find that the permission of one parent is sufficient for research to be conducted under Sec. 46.404 or Sec. 46.405. Where research is covered by Sec. 46.406 and Sec. 46.407 and permission is to be obtained from parents, both parents must give their permission unless one parent is deceased, unknown, incompetent, or not reasonably available, or when only one parent has legal responsibility for the care and custody of the child.

(c) In addition to the provisions for waiver contained in Sec. 46.116 of Subpart A, if the IRB determines that a research protocol is designed for conditions or for a subject population for which parental or guardian permission is not a reasonable requirement to protect the subjects (for example, neglected or abused children), it may waive the consent requirements in Subpart A of this part and paragraph (b) of this section, provided an appropriate mechanism for protecting the children who will participate as subjects in the research is substituted, and provided further that the waiver is not inconsistent with Federal, State, or local law.

The choice of an appropriate mechanism would depend upon the nature and purpose of the activities described in the protocol, the risk and anticipated benefit to the research subjects, and their age, maturity, status, and condition.

(d) Permission by parents or guardians shall be documented in accordance with and to the extent required by Sec. 46.117 of Subpart A.

(e) When the IRB determines that assent is required, it shall also determine whether and how assent must be documented.

Sec. 46.409 Wards.

(a) Children who are wards of the State or any other agency, institution, or entity can be included in research approved under Sec. 46.406 or Sec. 46.407 only if such research is:

(1) related to their status as wards; or

(2) conducted in schools, camps, hospitals, institutions, or similar settings in which the majority of children involved as subjects are not wards.

(b) If the research is approved under paragraph (a) of this section, the IRB shall require appointment of an advocate for each child who is a ward, in addition to any other individual acting on behalf of the child as guardian or in loco parentis. One individual may serve as advocate for more than one child. The advocate shall be an individual who has the background and experience to act in, and agrees to act in, the best interests of the child for the duration of the child's participation in the research and who is not associated in any way (except in the role as advocate or member of the IRB) with the research, the investigator(s), or the guardian organization.

GLOSSARY

Adverse Event - (AE) Any unfavorable or unintended event associated with a research study.

Adverse Event Reports - Investigator reports of all serious and adverse events, injury and deaths given to the sponsor, the IRB and the FDA.

Assurance - Renewable permit granted by a federal department to an institution to conduct research, can be given for individual or multiple projects.

Belmont Report - Ethical Principles and Guidelines for the Protection of Human Subjects of Research. Cornerstone document of ethical principles. Federal regulation of subject protection based on respect for persons, beneficence and justice.

Beneficence - Doing no harm, maximizing benefits while minimizing risks.

Case Report Forms - Study document of all data required by protocol on each subject.

Certified Clinical Research Coordinator - (CCRC) CRC with more than 2 years experience and with certification earned by passing required program and exam.

Clinical Research - Study of drug, biologic or device in human subjects with the intent to discover potential beneficial effects and/or determine its safety and efficacy. Also called clinical study and clinical investigation. Note that in this manual, this term is used in its narrow sense as used by the FDA. Thus, it does not encompass all the research that is carried out in the clinical setting (e.g., health services research).

Clinical Research Associate - (CRA) Person employed by the study sponsor or CRO to monitor a clinical study at all participating sites. See also, monitor.

Clinical Research Coordinator - (CRC) Site administer for the clinical study. Duties are delegated by the investigator. Also called research, study or healthcare coordinator, and data manager, research nurse or protocol nurse.

Clinical Study Materials - Study supplies (i.e., study test article, laboratory supplies case report forms) provided by the study sponsor to the investigator.

Common Rule - 1991 agreement to cover all federal-sponsored research by a common set of regulations.

Consent Form - Contains all relevant study information explained in lay terms and documents voluntary participation of subject. Presented to and signed by subject.

Contract Research Organization - (CRO) A person or an organization (commercial, academic or other) contracted by the sponsor to perform one or more of a sponsor's study-related duties and functions.

Data - Legally defined according to institution. Generally refers to recorded information regardless of form. Most institutions hold title to data while researchers have rights to access data.

Deception - Intentionally misleading or withholding information about nature of experiment.

Declaration of Helsinki - Statement of ethical principles first published by World Medical Association in 1964 to define rules for therapeutic and nontherapeutic research.

Documentation - All forms of records that describe or document study methods, conduct and results, including any adverse events and actions taken.

Drug or Device Accountability Records - (DAR) Required documentation for material accountability, quantity used and left over, and date of disposal.

Ethical Principles and Guidelines for the Protection of Human Subjects of Research - See Belmont Report.

Family Educational Rights and Privacy Act (FERPA)- Covers rights of parents of school children regarding reviewing, amending and disclosing educational records.

Food and Drug Administration - (FDA) Within DHHS. Enforces Food, Drug and Cosmetics Act and related federal public health laws. Grants IND, IDE, PMA and NDA approvals.

Food Drug and Cosmetic Act - (FD & C Act) States only drugs, biologics and devices proven safe and effective can be marketed.

FDA Form 1572 - List of commitments and conduct required by FDA for each investigator performing drug/biologics study. Also referred to as statement of investigator.

Good Clinical Practice - (GCP) International ethical and scientific quality standard for designing, conducting, monitoring, recording, auditing, analyzing and reporting studies. Insures that the data reported is credible and accurate and that subject's rights and confidentiality are protected.

Human Subject - A patient or healthy individual participating in a research study. A living individual about whom an investigator obtains private information or data through intervention or interaction.

Inclusion Criteria - A list of criteria that must be met by all study subjects.

Informed Consent - Information exchange including subject recruitment materials, verbal instructions, written materials, question and answer sessions and signature documenting consent with date. Subjects are given opportunity to choose involvement based on information, comprehension and voluntariness.

International Ethics Guidelines for Biomedical Research Involving Human Subjects - (CIOMS guidelines) Developed by the Council for International Organizations of Medical Sciences in 1982 to guide cross-cultural research.

Institution - Location of research. Retains ultimate responsibility for human subject regulation compliance.

Institutional Review Board - (IRB) Reviews research and consent forms to determine if rights and welfare of subjects are protected.

Investigational Device Exemption - (IDE) Exemption from FD & C Act to study investigational medical devices.

Investigational Materials - Test articles under clinical investigation.

Investigational New Drug Application - (IND) Exemption from FD & C Act to study investigational drug or biologic.

Investigator - Conducts and directs study. Carries ultimate responsibility for research. Is referred to as the principle investigator when acts as a leader for an investigational team. Also referred to as Clinical Investigator by the FDA.

Investigator-Sponsor - Individual with both responsibilities of initiating and conducting a clinical study.

Investigator's Brochure - Relevant clinical and nonclinical data compiled on the investigational drug, biologic or device being studied.

Kefauver-Harris Amendments - Amendment to FD & C Act that requires informed consent for experimental drugs.

Misconduct - Fabrication, falsification, plagiarism or other practices that seriously deviate from those accepted within scientific community for conducting and reporting research.

Monitor - Person employed by the sponsor or CRO who reviews study records to determine that a study is being conducted in accordance with the protocol. A monitor's duties may include, but are not limited to, helping to plan and initiate a study, and assessing the conduct of studies. Monitors work with the clinical research coordinator to check all data and documentation from the study. See also CRA.

Monitoring - Reviewing a clinical study, ensuring conduct, proper records and reports are performed as stated in the clinical protocol, standard operating procedures, GCP and by regulatory requirements.

Multiple Project Assurance - Permit given to institution for multiple federally funded research grants for a specified period of time. States institution retains responsibility for all research involving humans and that the institution must have an established IRB.

National Research Act - Act created the National Commission for Protection of Human Subjects of Biomedical and Behavioral research in 1974 and mandated review of studies by institutional review boards and subject protection by informed consent.

New Drug Application - (NDA) An FDA application to market a new drug in the United States.

National Institutes of Health - (NIH) Agency within DHHS that provides funding for research, conducts studies and funds multi-site national studies.

Nuremberg Code - Set of standards proclaimed following trial of Nazi doctors in 1947.

Office for Protection from Research Risk - (OPRR) Federal government office that issues Assurances and overseas compliance.

Patient - Individual seeking medical care.

Protection of Pupil Rights Amendment (PPRA) - Department of Education regulation that states that surveys, questionnaires and instructional materials for school children must be inspected by parents/guardians.

Protocol - Documentation of study objective, design, methods, statistical methods and organization. The term also includes amendments made to the original document.

Protocol Amendment - Changes or clarifications made in writing to the original protocol.

Recruitment - Act of enrolling subjects with the proper inclusion criteria.

Recruitment Period - Time allowed to recruit all subjects for a study.

Research - Systematic investigation designed to develop or contribute to generalizable knowledge. Includes Clinical Research.

Research Team - Investigator, subinvestigator and clinical research coordinator involved with study.

Risk-Benefit Ratio - Risk to individual subject vs potential benefits. Also called Risk-Benefit Analysis.

Safety Reports - FDA report required by investigator for any serious and unexpected adverse experience.

Serious Adverse Event - (SAE) Any event that results in death, a life threatening situation, hospitalization or prolonged hospitalization, disability, incapacity or a congenital anomaly/birth defect. Also called serious adverse drug reaction (serious ADR).

Single Project Assurance - Permit given to institution for single grant in compliance with government standards. See assurance.

Source Data - All information contained in original records and certified copies of results, observations or other facets required for the reconstruction and evaluation of the study that is contained in source documents.

Source Documentation - Location that information is first recorded including original documents, data and records.

Sponsor - Individual, company, institution or organization taking responsibility for initiation, management and financing of study.

Standard Operating Procedures - (SOP) Detailed, written procedures for the uniform performance of a function.

Subinvestigator - Helps design and conduct investigation at a study site.

Subject/Study Subject - Participant in a study. See Human Subject.

Telephone Report - Notification via telephone to the FDA of unexpected fatal or life threatening advent associated with clinical study.

Unexpected Adverse Drug Reaction - A reaction that is not consistent in nature or severity with study application.

Vulnerable Subjects - Group/individual that cannot give informed consent because of limited autonomy (e.g., children, mentally ill and prisoners). Also refers to subjects who may be unduly influenced to participate (e.g., students, subordinates and patients).

Well-being - Subject's physical and mental soundness.

Withdrawal Application - Investigator/sponsor letter to FDA requesting application withdrawal when no additional work is envisioned.

ABBREVIATIONS

Abbreviation	Term
AE	Adverse Event
AEC	Atomic Energy Commission
ACHRE	Advisory Committee on Human Radiation Experiments
AMA	American Medical Association
CCRC	Certified Clinical Research Coordinator
CDC	Centers for Disease Control and Prevention
CFR	Code of Federal Regulations
CIOMS	Council for International Organizations of Medical Sciences
CRC	Clinical Research Coordinator
CRO	Clinical Research Organization
DAR	Drug or Device Accountability Record
DHHS	Department of Health and Human Services
FDA	Food and Drug Administration
FD&C Act	Food, Drug, and Cosmetic Act
FERPA	Family Educational Rights and Privacy Act

Abbreviation	Term
GCP	Good Clinical Practice
ICH	International Conference on Harmonization
IDE	Investigational Device Exemption
IND	Investigational New Drug Application
IRB	Institutional Review Board
MPA	Multiple Project Assurance
NBAC	National Bioethics Advisory Commission
NCI	National Cancer Institute
NDA	New Drug Application
NIH	National Institutes of Health
NIOSH	National Institute for Occupational Safety & Health
OPRR	Office for Protection from Research Risks
ORI	Office of Research Integrity
PHS	Public Health Service
PI	Principal Investigator
PMA	Premarket Approval Application
PPRA	Protection of Pupil Rights Amendment
TBI	Total Body Irradiation

INDEX

Adverse Event 133, 172, 175

Advisory Committee on Human
Radiation Experiments 11

American Medical Association 81

Assurance 15, 16, 22, 25, 27, 28, 36, 39, 58, 71, 74, 192, 199, 200, 201

Atomic Energy Commission 12

Belmont Report 11, 15, 16, 24, 26, 29, 30, 92, 95

Case Report Forms 54, 65, 66, 65

Centers for Disease Control and Prevention 8

Clinical Research Associate 92

Clinical Research Coordinator..46, 92, 93

Code of Federal Regulations 29, 39, 92

Common Rule 11, 24, 25, 75

Consent Form 35, 166, 121, 152, 193, 206

Contract Research Organization ....

Declaration of Helsinki 4, 5, 6, 39, 158, 198

Department of Health and Human Services 24, 33, 37, 38, 1163, 171,
198, 207, 208, 211, 213

Drug or Device Accountability Record 63

Family Educational Rights and Privacy Act 18

FDA Form 1572...59

Food and Drug Administration (FDA).....7, 8, 11, 24-26, 28, 29, 30, 33,
34, 35, 37-39, 44, 57-62, 67-72, 80-83, 86, 89, 92, 93, 110, 111, 115,
117-120, 124, 125, 144, 147, 150, 151, 154, 157, 160-163, 171-180,
182, 190, 196, 198, 199

Food, Drug and Cosmetic Act 7, 38, 92

Good Clinical Practice (GCP)...............33, 38, 39, 40, 61, 62, 66, 92, 93

Informed Consent......1, 4, 5, 6, 8, 11, 12, 15, 20, 22, 25, 26, 34, 35, 37
40, 42, 48, 51, 60-62, 65-67, 75, 76, 91, 100, 102, 105, 112-116, 121,
122, 124, 133, 139, 140, 143, 149, 150, 152, 156, 159, 160, 182-186,
188-190, 193, 195, 196, 202-206, 209, 210

Institutional Review Board (IRB) .7, 11, 15, 20, 24, 25-30, 34-36, 38, 39, 42, 45, 51-54, 60-64, 66-71, 74-76, 92, 93, 106, 112-122, 128-130, 133, 139, 141, 149, 150, 151, 153, 156, 178, 180, 183, 187-212, 214, 218

International Conference on Harmonization..38

Investigational Device Exemption........35, 111, 117, 124, 127, 128, 160, 174, 179

Investigational New Drug Application 35, 110, 111, 115, 117, 124, 127, 128, 160, 174, 179

Monitor..1,5, 25, 27, 28, 35, 38, 39, 47, 53, 54, 60-62, 66, 68, 82, 110, 123, 125, 127, 129, 130, 133, 140, 148-150, 156, 178, 180, 184, 186-190, 195, 203, 209, 214, 120-156, 158, 159, 161, 178-196, 200, 204

Multiple Project Assurance 16, 27

National Bioethics Advisory Commission....................................11, 13, 20

National Institutes of Health (NIH) 37, 47, 61, 85, 92, 198, 200, 202

National Research Act...11, 16, 24

New Drug Application 35, 110, 111, 115, 117, 124-128, 160, 174, 179

Nuremburg Code 5

Office for Protection from Research Risk...............27, 92, 198, 200, 202

Office of Research Integrity...........................31, 32, 37, 38, 92

Premarket Approval Application 179, 194

Principal Investigator (PI) 44, 46, 63, 64, 212

Protection of Pupil Rights Amendment...................................19

Public Health Service 8, 30, 37, 110, 112, 118, 119, 124, 125, 157, 161, 163

Sponsor.........11, 12, 15, 24-27, 35-39, 42, 45, 47, 53-64, 66-72, 79-89, 110-113, 115, 119

Total Body Irradiation 12

Vulnerable Subjects..17, 47, 76, 106

PROTECTING STUDY VOLUNTEERS EXAMINATION (PART 1)

True/False

1. It is appropriate to forgo subject protection if the benefit to science and society is great enough.

    A. True

    B. False

2. An investigator is required to prepare and maintain adequate and accurate records and case histories for all clinical trial subjects.

    A. True

    B. False

3. Research must be reviewed at least annually by the IRB to prevent suspension of the study.

    A. True

    B. False

4. Research that is approved by the IRB for adults is automatically approved for children.

    A. True

    B. False

5. Adverse consequences resulting from an investigator's violation of ethical research practices only impact that particular investigator.

    A. True

    B. False

6. Both the investigator and the sponsor have responsibilities for drug/device accountability.

    A. True

    B. False

7. It is a criminal offense to have signed the FORM FDA 1572 form if commitments made within the document are ignored.

    A. True

    B. False

8. The investigator is not required to report a serious adverse event to the sponsor if it is reported to the IRB.
    A. True
    B. False

9. Maintenance of adequate and accurate case histories for study subjects includes documentation that informed consent was obtained prior to a subject's participation in the study.
    A. True
    B. False

10. Professional judgment is required throughout the research process.
    A. True
    B. False

11. The only circumstance in which an investigator can deviate from the protocol without prior IRB approval is for safety reasons.
    A. True
    B. False

12. The investigator has primary responsibility for conducting the study, supervising all personnel, and for protecting the rights, safety, and welfare of research subjects.
    A. True
    B. False

13. Research that is exempt from federal regulations may require review by someone other than the investigator to verify exempt status.
    A. True
    B. False

14. Women of childbearing potential may be routinely excluded from participating in research.
    A. True
    B. False

15. Retaliation against a 'whistle-blower' may be construed as an act of misconduct.
    A. True
    B. False

16. Investigators bear the ultimate responsibility for the safety and welfare of their human subjects.
    A. True
    B. False

Multiple Choice

17. **Advertising for study subjects must:**
    A. make claims of safety and efficacy
    B. be approved by the IRB
    C. be limited to posters and pamphlets
    D. all of the above
    E. none of the above

18. **The following items are considered during IRB review of a study.**
    A. consent process
    B. the risks to the subjects
    C. recruitment methods
    D. all of the above
    E. none of the above

19. **What is included in the official definition of scientific misconduct?**
    A. fabrication, falsification, plagiarism or other practices that significantly deviate from accepted standards
    B. negligence and errors
    C. incompetence or negative results
    D. differences in interpretation
    E. none of the above

20. **Which of the following best describes the consent process?**
    A. the subject signing the consent form
    B. an information exchange between subject and investigator before, during and sometimes even after participation
    C. ascertaining that the subject has comprehended the information in the consent form
    D. providing a setting free of coercion and undue influence
    E. the subject reading and signing the consent form

21. **A risk factor for research subjects in a study may be:**
    A. psychological
    B. economic
    C. legal
    D. social
    E. all of the above

22. Regarding the Syphilis study:
    A. from the beginning, the intent was to withhold treatment on a long term basis
    B. the subjects were kept informed about their disease
    C. it was an example that scientists with the best intentions sometimes forget that people's rights must be protected
    D. all of the above
    E. none of the above

23. As defined in the Belmont Report, <u>beneficence</u> relates to this general rule:
    A. always get consent
    B. maximize possible benefits and minimize risks
    C. burdens of research should not be imposed unduly
    D. none of the above
    E. all of the above

24. As defined in the Belmont Report, the principle of <u>respect for persons</u> includes:
    A. the requirement to acknowledge autonomy
    B. excluding women from clinical trials
    C. the requirement to protect those with diminished autonomy
    D. a and c
    E. all of the above

25. The IRB has the authority to:
    A. disapprove a new research proposal
    B. require modifications to an ongoing study
    C. disallow proposed changes to an active protocol
    D. all of the above
    E. none of the above

26. What actions must an investigator take to implement an amendment in a study design/protocol?
    A. obtain IRB approval of the amendment before implementing the change
    B. if the amendment includes modification of the consent form, get IRB approval prior to use
    C. if directed by the IRB, obtain new consent from subjects already enrolled
    D. all of the above
    E. none of the above

27. **Investigators who also take on the role of sponsors**
    A. must comply with the responsibilities of both investigators and sponsors
    B. only must comply with investigator responsibilities
    C. only must comply with sponsor responsibilities
    D. all of the above
    E. none of the above

28. **What are two protections for human subjects in current federal regulations?**
    A. payment to subjects and right to advertise
    B. informed consent and payment to subjects
    C. informed consent and IRB review
    D. absolute confidentiality and payment to subjects
    E. all of the above

29. **What actions can the FDA take against investigators who violate regulations?**
    A. criminal actions
    B. injunctions
    C. fines
    D. all of the above
    E. none of the above

30. **Which group is <u>not</u> representative of a vulnerable population for which special federal regulations have been written?**
    A. pregnant woman
    B. deceased patients
    C. children
    D. prisoners
    E. b and c

PROTECTING STUDY VOLUNTEERS EXAMINATION (PART 2)

Please read the following case studies and answer the corresponding questions.

Case Study – 1
Scenario #1

Drug "Seizure-stop" is a marketed product in tablet form for oral administration to treat epileptic seizures in patients over 12 years old.

An IND would be required for research with Drug "Seizure-stop" in:

1. Following reformulation in the hospital pharmacy, the drug will be administered intravenously to adults with moderate epilepsy.
   A. True
   B. False

2. Neonates with intractable seizures
   A. True
   B. False

Scenario #2

Device "Graft-ease" has an IDE as an aortic graft prosthesis, but is not approved for marketing.

3. IRB approval is required for use in aortic repair in non-emergency situations
   A. True
   B. False

4. A new IDE is not required for studying "Graft-ease" in other arteries, for example in renal (kidney) artery disease
   A. True
   B. False

Scenario #3

Compound Z has well-documented physiological effects in animal studies which you would like to explore. It is available in powder form from a local chemical supplier. Compound Z is not approved for any use by FDA.

An IND is required to use Compound Z in:

5. **Healthy human volunteers**
   A. True
   B. False

6. **Terminally ill patients**
   A. True
   B. False

Case Study – 2

A placebo-controlled, multi-center trial of a new combination therapy for weight loss is being conducted and you are the principal investigator for one of the sites. The two drugs being studied are both marketed products, and both are known to cause heart palpitations when prescribed alone. There are no other cardiovascular side effects listed for these drugs. The study design requires that the subjects start an exercise plan for two weeks prior to being randomized to the study drugs.

1. **A 65 year old man whom you enrolled with consent has a heart attack on the second day of the exercise plan. The subject has not been randomized and has not received either of the study medications. This event should be reported to your IRB.**
   A. True
   B. False

2. **After several reports of clinically significant arrhythmia, the protocol is amended to exclude patients with a history of cardiovascular disease. The consent form is amended to include the risk of significant irregular heartbeats. These changes do not have to be approved by the IRB because they are minor and add protections.**
   A. True
   B. False

Case Study – 3

Informed consent is a major human subject protection mechanism and investigators must be sensitive to all aspects of the process. Research protocols and model consent forms are sometimes provided by sponsors of research. Examples include industry-sponsored drug/device studies, NIH-supported cancer study groups, and some foundation grants. The model consent forms may contain all of the eight required element sections (Purpose, Risks, Benefits, Alternatives, Injury Compensation, Confidentiality, Contacts, and Voluntary Participation Statement), however, investigators at study sites are expected to review and modify these models as necessary to account for local conditions.

Scenario #1

A proposed research study will recruit all critically ill patients in the local emergency room (ER) over a six-month period. ER nurses will obtain consent for the study. Follow-up visits will occur as will review of medical records and billing information.

1. To avoid undue inducement/pressure, the method in which consent is sought should provide adequate time for the subject to make a decision
    A. True
    B. False

2. The principal investigator is always ultimately responsible for ensuring that consent is properly obtained, however the PI may delegate, to appropriately qualified and trained persons, part or all of the consent discussion
    A. True
    B. False

3. This study will obviously involve vulnerable populations such as individuals with cognitive disorders and critically/terminally ill patients. Children and pregnant women are likely candidates as well. Additional human subject protections that may be applicable to this study include:
    A. use of consent witnesses/monitors in the ER
    B. having the study reviewed by local consultants/advocates
    C. formally renewing/re-verifying consent at a later time
    D. all of the above
    E. none of the above

4. Because children will be enrolled in the study, adequate provision for soliciting the assent of the child-subject must be made in addition to obtaining parental permission.

   A. True
   B. False

5. The study design and the investigators procedures and facilities must be adequate to protect against unintentional releases of identifiable information gained from the medical and billing records.

   A. True
   B. False

Scenario #2

FDA guidance instructs that payments to subjects are not to be considered by the IRB as a benefit, but rather as an incentive or inducement to subjects. The model consent contains this wording: "Payment for participation will be given upon completion of all six phases of the study. Because partial data is not valuable to us, if you withdraw, you will receive no payment."

6. To avoid undue inducement (pressuring subjects to continue when they otherwise might have withdrawn), the protocol and this wording should be changed to provide a prorated amount, based upon phases completed at the time of withdrawal.

   A. True
   B. False

7. If partial data is not useful for analysis, almost all of the payment could be offered to subjects as a completion bonus, despite considerable inconveniences to the subjects throughout the six study phases.

   A. True
   B. False

8. If advertisements will be used to recruit subjects for this study, the ads must receive IRB approval before they are used.

   A. True
   B. False

Scenario #3

You are presented with a model consent document for a study that, while listing paragraph after paragraph of potential health risks, leaves out any discussion of likely economic impact and quality of life issues. The consent form contains the following wording, "While the risks are considerable, so are the benefits. This drug combination has been shown to be safe and effective in treating your condition. Even if you don't benefit directly, many terminally ill patients will live longer because of the knowledge gained in this study."

9. Leaving out most of the risks from the consent form would probably result in higher enrollments. This is acceptable if the important ones are discussed verbally.
   A. True
   B. False

10. Regarding risks and benefits of research:
    A. presenting both risks and benefits is based upon the Belmont principles
    B. weighing of risks and benefits is important in the subject's decision to enroll in a study
    C. accurate information that does not understate risks or overstate benefits is essential
    D. all of the above
    E. none of the above

11. The wording used in the model should be changed to avoid overstating benefits.
    A. True
    B. False

12. Reasonably foreseeable risks, including those not health-related such as economic risks, should be added to the consent form/consent process so that subjects may consider them in making a decision.
    A. True
    B. False

Notes

Notes

Notes